Paediatric Immediate Life Support

3rd Edition September 2016
Reprinted in July 2018

ISBN 978-1-903812-34-1

Paediatric Immediate Life Support

3rd Edition September 2016 – Reprinted in July 2018

Editors

Sophie Skellett

Sue Hampshire

Sarah Mitchell

Liz Norris

Contributors

Robert Bingham

Fiona Clements

Karen Cooper

Mike Coren

Sue Hampshire

Ben Lakin

Ian Maconochie

Ian McDougall

Sarah Mitchell

Liz Norris

Ruchi Sinha

Sophie Skellett

Felicity Todd

Mark Woolcock

Mark Worrall

Jonathan Wyllie

Deborah Zeitlin

Acknowledgements

We thank and acknowledge the members of the ERC 2015 Guidelines Writing Group who have contributed directly or indirectly to this PILS Manual.

We thank Mark Sedge for taking the photographs for this manual and the models and their parents for giving up their time to help with these. We also thank Paul Wood for his help with the final preparation for printing.

Printed on responsibly sourced environmentally friendly paper made with elemental chlorine free fibre from legal and sustainably managed forests.

Finally, we would like to thank all the course centres and instructors for their contributions to the Paediatric Immediate Life Support course.

Published by Resuscitation Council (UK)
5th Floor, Tavistock House North, Tavistock Square, London WC1H 9HR
Tel: 020 7388 4678   Fax: 020 7383 0773   E-mail: enquiries@resus.org.uk   Website: www.resus.org.uk

Printed by: All About Print
Tel: 020 7205 4022   Email: hello@allaboutprint.co.uk   Website: www.allaboutprint.co.uk

The Resuscitation Council (UK) guidelines are adapted from the European Resuscitation Council guidelines and have been developed using a process accredited by The National Institute for Health and Care Excellence. The UK guidelines are consistent with the European guidelines but include minor modifications to reflect the needs of the National Health Service.

This Paediatric Immediate Life Support (PILS) manual is written by the Resuscitation Council (UK) EPALS Subcommittee and forms part of the resources for the Resuscitation Council (UK) PILS course, which is delivered in accredited course centres throughout the UK.

Paediatric Immediate Life Support

Introduction to the course

The Paediatric Immediate Life Support (PILS) course aims to provide healthcare staff with the requisite knowledge and skills to enable them to:

- understand the structured ABCDE approach that facilitates rapid recognition of seriously ill children

- provide appropriate initial treatment interventions to prevent cardiorespiratory arrest

- treat children in respiratory or cardiorespiratory arrest until the arrival of a resuscitation team or more experienced assistance

- become members of a paediatric resuscitation team.

This publication is predominantly based on the resuscitation of children in the acute hospital setting. However, the same principles apply to the resuscitation of children in any clinical setting (e.g. community hospital).

The PILS course teaches how to recognise the seriously ill child, as well as how to start cardiopulmonary resuscitation in the clinical setting. This includes delivery of effective ventilation and chest compressions. Only those medications that might be required in the first few minutes of cardiopulmonary resuscitation are discussed.

The actual course is delivered as hands-on practical skill stations, workshops and simulations, with as little information as possible presented in lecture format. This is to maximise the time spent in developing skills in the structured ABCDE assessment. This approach should not only ensure early recognition of the child at risk of, but also prevent progression to, respiratory or cardiorespiratory arrest. If respiratory or cardiorespiratory arrest should occur, the other skills practised on the PILS course are those that are most likely to successfully resuscitate the child.

Glossary

- AED — Automated external defibrillator
- BLS — Basic life support
- BMV — Bag-mask ventilation
- BP — Blood pressure
- CO — Cardiac output
- CO_2 — Carbon dioxide
- CPR — Cardiopulmonary resuscitation
- CRT — Capillary refill time
- ECG — Electrocardiogram
- EMS — Emergency medical service (e.g. ambulance service)
- FEV — Forced expiratory volume
- FiO_2 — Fraction of inspired oxygen
- HR — Heart rate
- H — Hours
- IM — Intramuscular
- IO — Intraosseous
- IV — Intravenous
- O_2 — Oxygen
- $PaCO_2$ — Partial pressure of arterial carbon dioxide
- EPALS — European paediatric advanced life support
- Min — Minutes
- PEA — Pulseless electrical activity
- PEEP — Positive end expiratory pressure
- PEF — Peak expiratory flow
- PICU — Paediatric intensive care unit
- ROSC — Return of spontaneous circulation
- RR — Respiratory rate
- SaO_2 — Arterial oxygen saturation
- S — Seconds
- SpO_2 — Peripheral arterial oxygen saturation from an oximeter probe
- SV — Stroke volume
- SVR — Systemic vascular resistance
- SVT — Supraventricular tachycardia
- Tidal volume — Volume of each breath
- VF — Ventricular fibrillation
- pVT — pulseless VT
- VT — Ventricular tachycardia
- $<$ — Less than
- $\leq$ — Less than or equal to
- $>$ — Greater than
- $\geq$ — Greater than or equal to

Throughout this publication the masculine parts of speech (he, him and his) are used generically.

Contents

Introduction to Paediatric Life Support

Contents

- **The differences between primary and secondary cardiorespiratory arrest**
- **Outcomes from respiratory and cardiorespiratory arrest in children**
- **Basic anatomy and physiology of an infant or child's airway, breathing, and circulation**
- **How differences in anatomy and physiology influence resuscitation of a seriously ill child**

Learning outcomes

To enable you to:

- **Understand how the aetiologies of cardiorespiratory arrest in children differ from those in adults**
- **Understand the probable outcome of primary and secondary cardiorespiratory arrest**
- **Appreciate why specific anatomical and physiological properties of infants and young children influence their clinical management**

Aetiologies of cardiorespiratory arrest

The aetiology of cardiorespiratory arrest in children differs from adults. This is due to anatomical, physiological and pathological differences which alter throughout childhood.

Primary cardiorespiratory arrest is a sudden acute event which occurs without warning. It is commonly due to a cardiac arrhythmia reflecting intrinsic heart disease. Successful outcome is generally dependent on rapid defibrillation, as the most common arrhythmias encountered in primary cardiorespiratory arrest victims are ventricular fibrillation (VF) or pulseless ventricular tachycardia (pVT). Every minute of delay until defibrillation results in the number of successful cases returning to spontaneous circulation decreasing by approximately 10%.

Primary cardiorespiratory arrest is most common in adults but can occur in older children or children with congenital heart disease. The most common aetiology of cardiorespiratory arrest in children overall is secondary to other intercurrent illness.

This secondary cardiorespiratory arrest is usually due to hypoxia and reflects the limit of the body's ability to compensate for the effects of underlying illness or injury. Severe tissue hypoxia causes myocardial dysfunction, resulting in profound bradycardia which typically deteriorates to asystole or pulseless electrical activity (PEA). Both PEA and asystole are associated with a poor outcome.

Secondary cardiorespiratory arrest is rarely a sudden event, but follows a progressive deterioration. As respiratory and circulatory failure worsen (Figure 1.1), the body initially activates adaptive physiological responses aimed at limiting the effects of the deterioration on vital organs (compensated respiratory or circulatory failure). These adaptive responses will result in signs and symptoms that can be recognised, thereby providing an opportunity to intervene before further deterioration to cardiorespiratory arrest.

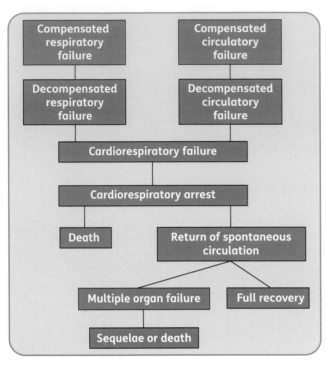

Figure 1.1 Consequences of progressive respiratory or circulatory failure

Outcome from secondary cardiorespiratory arrest

The outcome from secondary cardiorespiratory arrest is poor. Severe tissue hypoxia occurring before the heart stops means that all the vital organs are potentially seriously compromised; the heart finally arrests as a result of severe myocardial hypoxia.

Even if a return of spontaneous circulation (ROSC) is achieved, morbidity and mortality remains high. Successful resuscitation from secondary cardiorespiratory arrest for out-of-hospital events is low (4.5–7.6% survival) and less than 5% of children will survive without neurological sequelae. In-hospital cardiac arrest (IHCA) results are better with 70% ROSC rate but many children succumb to severe organ injury (e.g. brain, kidney) or multi-system organ failure, 48–72 h post arrest; overall for IHCA 35–40% children will survive to discharge. Resuscitation from respiratory arrest, when there is still cardiac output, is associated with much better (70–90%) good quality, long-term survival.

Anatomical and physiological considerations

The underlying anatomical and physiological differences between infants, young children and adults largely account for the difference in aetiology of cardiorespiratory arrest.

The key differences will be considered in order of management priority based on the mnemonic ABCDE.

> A **Airway**
>
> B **Breathing**
>
> C **Circulation**
>
> D **Disability (mental status)**
>
> E **Exposure**

Airway

The infant/young child has an airway that is proportionately narrower and more susceptible to oedema and swelling than the adult. The absolute diameter of the airway is also smaller, and therefore respiratory infections account for a significantly higher level of morbidity and mortality in young children.

Relationship between head and neck

The infant's head is large in relation to the rest of their body. Since the occiput is protuberant, the head tends to flex on the neck when the infant is placed in a supine position. This leads to potential obstruction of the airway when the conscious level is reduced. With increasing age, the child's head becomes smaller in relation to their thorax, the neck lengthens and the larynx becomes more resistant to external pressure as tissues become less compliant.

Face and mouth

The infant's face is small and therefore the sizing of facemasks needs to be accurate otherwise it is difficult to achieve an effective seal. Additionally, pressure to the eyes can lead to damage and reflex bradycardia.

Inside the small mouth the tongue is relatively large. This combination means that airway obstruction is more likely in the unconscious infant/young child. The floor of the mouth is easily compressible; care is necessary to avoid compressing the soft tissues under the mandible to prevent airway obstruction when performing airway manoeuvres.

Nose and pharynx

The infant is a preferential nasal breather for the first six months or so of life. As a result, anything that causes nasal obstruction (e.g. anatomical abnormalities such as choanal atresia, copious secretions, nasogastric tubes or tapes) can lead to increased work of breathing and respiratory compromise.

The larynx

The epiglottis in infants is larger and floppier than in adults. This means that it is vulnerable to damage by airway devices and manoeuvres.

The larynx is higher in the infant compared to the older child and adult (where it is level with C5–6). Until about 8 years, the child's larynx is funnel shaped, with its narrowest segment at the level of the cricoid cartilage, as opposed to the older child/adult, who has a larynx that is cylindrical in shape. The anatomical variations have the following practical implications:

- Blind finger sweeps to remove a foreign body must not be performed in young children with partial airway obstruction as these may convert a partial into a complete obstruction. The foreign body can become impacted into the narrowest part of the larynx (i.e. at the cricoid cartilage).

- The relatively large tongue may create airway obstruction as the epiglottis and larynx are higher in the neck.

- Control of the large tongue with a laryngoscope blade may be difficult.

- The high position of the larynx in an infant creates a sharp angle between the oropharynx and the glottis. Direct visualisation of the glottis with the laryngoscope is therefore difficult. It may be easier to use a straight blade rather than a curved blade to obtain a view, particularly in infants up to three months of age.

Breathing

Physiological considerations

Infants and small children have a relatively small resting lung volume and hence a low oxygen reserve. In addition, they have a high rate of oxygen consumption. This combination results in very rapid falls in blood oxygen levels in respiratory compromise.

Spontaneous tidal volume stays constant throughout life at 4–6 mL kg^{-1}. It can be qualitatively assessed by auscultation of the chest, listening to air entry in the upper and lower zones of both sides of the chest.

Mechanics of breathing

As they age, the mechanics of children's breathing changes. The infant has ribs that are cartilaginous and pliable, while their intercostal muscles are weak and relatively ineffective. The main muscle of respiration is the diaphragm. During inspiration, the diaphragm descends towards the abdomen, generating a negative pressure, which draws air into the upper airway and the lungs. Mechanical impedance to the contraction of the diaphragm (e.g. gastric distension, intestinal obstruction) will result in ineffective ventilation, as will any obstruction of the airway (e.g. bronchiolitis, asthma or foreign body aspiration).

In older children, the more developed intercostal muscles contribute significantly to the mechanics of breathing. The ribs ossify and act as a secure anchor for the muscles, as well as forming a more rigid structure that is less likely to collapse in respiratory distress. In children above 5 years the presence of significant intercostal recession should therefore be considered as an ominous sign and indicative of serious respiratory compromise.

Respiratory rate

Normal respiration requires minimal effort and the resting respiratory rate varies with age. The infant has a relatively high metabolic rate, oxygen consumption and carbon dioxide production, which is the main reason for their increased respiratory rates (Table 1.1). The respiratory rate also increases with agitation, anxiety and the presence of fever, therefore a record of respiratory rate as it changes over time is more useful than a single value.

Table 1.1 Respiratory rate ranges by age	
Age (years)	Respiratory rate (breaths min^{-1})
< 1	30–40
1–2	26–34
2–5	24–30
5–12	20–24
> 12	12–20

Circulation

The circulating volume of the newborn is 80 mL kg^{-1} and decreases with age to 60–70 mL kg^{-1} in adulthood. This means that the total circulating volume of an infant is very small (e.g. 240 mL in a newborn of 3 kg and 480 mL in a 6 month old with a weight of 6 kg). Relatively small losses can be a significantly high percentage of their total circulating volume; this is why apparently minor diarrhoeal illnesses can result in considerable morbidity and even mortality in infants and young children.

Heart rate

Stroke volume (i.e. the amount of blood ejected with each contraction of the heart) is relatively small in infancy (1.5 mL kg^{-1} at birth) and increases along with heart size. However, the cardiac output relative to body weight is higher than at any other stage of life (300 mL kg^{-1} min^{-1}, decreasing to 100 mL kg^{-1} min^{-1} in adolescence and 70–80 mL kg^{-1} min^{-1} in adults).

Cardiac output is the product of stroke volume and heart rate, and so the high cardiac outputs in infants and young children are primarily achieved by rapid heart rates (Table 1.2).

Table 1.2 Heart rate ranges (beats min^{-1})			
Age	Mean	Awake	Deep sleep
Newborn – 3 months	140	85–205	80–140
3 months – 2 years	130	100–180	75–160
2–10 years	80	60–140	60–90
> 10 years	75	60–100	50–90

Table 1.3 Blood pressure ranges by age systolic and mean				
Age	Systolic BP 5th centile mmHg	Systolic BP 50th centile mmHg	Mean BP 5th centile mmHg	Mean BP 50th centile mmHg
0–1 month	50	60	35	45
1–12 months	70	80	40	55
1–10 years	70 + 2 x age in years	90 + 2 x age in years	40 + 1.5 x age (years)	55 + 1.5 x age (years)
15 years	90	120	65	80

Since cardiac output is directly related to the heart rate, bradycardia is a serious event and should be treated vigorously.

Systemic vascular resistance increases as the child ages and this is reflected in the changes seen in systolic blood pressure (BP) ranges, however, mean blood pressure values may more accurately reflect tissue perfusion in shocked states (Table 1.3).

Disability

The limited communication skills of infants and children have to be considered when attempting to assess neurological status. There is a tendency for ill children to regress to behaviour more befitting a younger child, especially if they are anxious or in pain.

Effective pain control, empathy and appropriate language are therefore all essential factors when dealing with children. The presence of parents or other significant adults may help to alleviate many communication difficulties, as well as helping to allay fear and anxiety.

A rapid assessment of the child's conscious level can be obtained by determining the AVPU score (Chapter 2). Additionally, assessment of pupil size and reaction, and the child's posture, muscle tone and any focal signs should be noted to determine neurological status.

Exposure

To ensure that no significant clinical information is missed, examine the child fully by exposing their body. Appropriate measures to minimise heat loss (especially in infants) and respect dignity must be adopted at all times. The core body temperature should also be recorded and if necessary, appropriate measures to normalise it initiated.

Weight estimation

Medications are prescribed based on a child's body weight. In the emergency situation, it is often impractical to weigh the child and it is important to have an alternative method of estimating weight as accurately as possible. Examples include the Broselow tape or the Sandell tape, which relates the length of the child to their body weight, or centile charts that estimate weight against age.

An infant weighs approximately 3 kg at birth and 10 kg at one year of age.

For the age group between 1 and 10 years the following formula provides an approximation of weight:

$$\text{Weight (kg)} = (\text{Age in years} + 4) \times 2$$

The simplicity of this formula facilitates recollection under pressure and although the actual weight of obese children will be underestimated, drug dosage is usually based on lean body mass rather than actual mass. The action of intravenous resuscitation drugs in particular depends on plasma concentration so drug dosage based on lean body mass is appropriate.

Whatever method is used to establish the body weight of a child it is essential that healthcare professionals are sufficiently familiar and competent in its use to be able to utilise it quickly and accurately. When employing weight based calculations do not administer a dose greater than the adult dose.

Summary learning

- **Children are more likely to suffer a secondary, rather than a primary cardiorespiratory arrest.**

- **Successful resuscitation from respiratory arrest, is associated with 70–90% survival.**

- **Survival from cardiorespiratory arrest is considerably less (< 5% out of hospital and approximately 35–40% in hospital).**

- **The mnemonic ABCDE is the basis of both the assessment and the management of seriously ill/injured children.**

My key take-home messages from this chapter

Recognition and initial management of the seriously ill child

Contents

- **Identifying the signs and symptoms of respiratory, circulatory and cardiorespiratory failure**
- **Parameters assessed during the ABCDE approach**
- **Using the ABCDE assessment to institute initial management of the airway breathing and circulation**

Learning outcomes

To enable you to:

- **Appreciate the importance of early recognition of the seriously ill child**
- **Understand the importance of the structured ABCDE approach to rapidly identify potential respiratory, circulatory and/or central neurological failure in the seriously ill child**
- **Use the structured ABCDE approach to prioritise and assess effectiveness of initial management strategies**

Early recognition of the seriously ill child

In children, cardiorespiratory arrest is usually due to hypoxia, reflecting the end of the body's ability to compensate for the effects of underlying illness or injury. The initial problem may originate from the airway, breathing or circulation. Irrespective of the primary aetiology, cardiorespiratory arrest in children is rarely a sudden event, but a progressive deterioration from combined respiratory and circulatory failure.

Early recognition and effective management of respiratory and/or circulatory failure will prevent the majority of paediatric cardiorespiratory arrests and thus reduce morbidity and mortality. It can also help identify children for whom cardiorespiratory resuscitation may be inappropriate which can help facilitate suitable palliative care.

The principles outlined in this chapter apply to the seriously ill child in all environments, (i.e. the acute hospital setting or out-of-hospital). Use of the structured ABCDE approach (detailed later in this chapter) helps to ensure that potentially life-threatening problems are identified and managed in order of their priority.

A: Airway problems

A review of practical airway management procedures is provided in Chapter 4.

Causes of airway obstruction

Airway obstruction can be partial or complete, sudden or insidious, progressive or recurrent. Respiratory rate and work of breathing generally increase in airway obstruction. When assessing airway patency, **chest movement does not guarantee that the airway is clear.** Air entry needs to be assessed by looking, listening and feeling for air movement, and by chest auscultation.

Initially, airway obstruction is often partial but can lead to respiratory failure, exhaustion, secondary apnoea and eventually hypoxic brain damage. Additionally, partial airway obstruction can rapidly become total, and result in cardiorespiratory arrest.

Congenital abnormalities such as choanal atresia or Pierre-Robin syndrome can be initially managed by use of an appropriate airway adjunct to open the airway and buy time, prior to definitive treatment.

Depression of the central nervous system can cause loss of airway control as protective upper airway reflexes and muscle tone are lost. This may be compounded in the infant due to the age related anatomical features. The pronounced occiput and short neck causes head flexion in the supine position and, together with the proportionately large tongue, can quickly lead to airway obstruction in the unconscious infant.

Causes of central nervous system depression include hypoxia following decompensated respiratory or circulatory failure, head trauma, metabolic disorders (e.g. hypoglycaemia, inborn errors of metabolism), hypercapnia, alcohol and medications (e.g. opiates, benzodiazepines). Airway obstruction due to these causes may not be accompanied by tachypnoea or increased work of breathing.

Table 2.1 Causes of airway obstruction

- Congenital abnormality (e.g. choanal atresia, Pierre-Robin syndrome)
- Secretions (e.g. vomit, blood)
- Respiratory tract infections (swelling or mucus secretions)
- Pharyngeal swelling (e.g. oedema, infection)
- Epiglottitis
- Laryngotracheobronchitis (croup)
- Nasal feeding tubes
- Oxygen delivery devices (e.g. nasal cannulae)
- Foreign body (e.g. food, toy, orthodontic appliances)
- Central nervous system depression (loss of muscle tone)
- Trauma (facial or throat)

Recognition of upper airway obstruction

Airway obstruction may be demonstrated by difficulty in breathing and/or increased respiratory effort. In a conscious child there may be visible distress. There may be additional respiratory noises, such as inspiratory stridor, if the obstruction is partial, whereas respiration will be silent in total obstruction.

Management of upper airway obstruction

The treatment of partial airway obstruction is to maintain airway patency and ensure that it does not become totally occluded. This may be achieved by head positioning, clearance of any secretions or foreign bodies, and summoning further assistance as indicated.

In patients with airway obstruction, delivery of supplemental oxygen is advised as early as possible, to minimise the potential effects of hypoxia.

The conscious child will usually adopt a position that optimises airway patency. If the child is stable, and deterioration is considered unlikely, he should be left with his parents/carers who can help administer oxygen and minimise stress and anxiety. Feeding should be avoided, and any fever treated to reduce increased metabolic demand. **If there is a decreased level of consciousness, airway compromise must be assumed.** The management priorities are to get more help whilst safeguarding the airway and preventing complications such as aspiration of gastric contents, by placing the child in the recovery position or supporting the head-up position.

Basic airway opening manoeuvres (e.g. head tilt and chin lift or jaw thrust) should be used. Adjuncts such as oro/nasopharyngeal airways can also be used until more experienced help is available. Advanced emergency airway management may involve insertion of a tracheal tube, laryngeal mask airway (LMA) or cricothyroidotomy, although the latter will only provide temporary oxygenation until a definitive airway can be achieved.

B: Breathing problems

In all seriously ill or injured children, the priority is for the appropriate management of the airway and ventilation (breathing).

Causes of breathing (respiratory) problems

Respiratory failure can result from acute or chronic breathing inadequacy. The underlying problem may be due to lung pathology (i.e. congenital or acquired diseases or trauma) or have a non-respiratory origin (e.g. circulatory failure, metabolic disorder, neurological problem).

The respiratory rate can be classified as abnormal if it is too rapid (tachypnoea), too slow (bradypnoea) or absent (apnoea). Respiratory distress is a clinical syndrome which reflects increased work of breathing, often associated with attempts to increase tidal volume and can be associated with either tachypnoea or bradypnoea.

As the work of breathing increases, an increased proportion of the cardiac output is diverted to the respiratory muscles with a consequent increase in the amount of carbon dioxide produced.

Ultimately, if the respiratory system is unable to provide sufficient oxygen for tissue requirements, anaerobic metabolism occurs and respiratory acidosis is complicated by metabolic acidosis.

Recognition of respiratory failure

From a physiological viewpoint, respiratory failure is usually defined as failure of the respiratory system to maintain an arterial oxygen level (PaO_2) > 9 kPa with 21% inspired O_2 (air) or/and arterial carbon dioxide level ($PaCO_2$) of < 6.5 kPa. This definition requires arterial blood gas analysis, which can be difficult to obtain in children.

A PaO_2 of 9 kPa corresponds approximately to a peripheral oxygen saturation (SpO_2) of 90%.

A child with respiratory distress may be able to maintain their arterial blood gases values within relatively normal limits by increasing their respiratory effort. It is therefore important to evaluate whether the child's situation is stable or if decompensation to respiratory failure is imminent. This evaluation requires knowledge of the signs and symptoms of respiratory distress and/or respiratory failure. When the compensatory mechanisms fail, deterioration is rapid and imminent cardiorespiratory arrest must be anticipated.

Warning signs of respiratory failure are:

- decreased level of consciousness

- hypotonia

- decreased respiratory effort

- cyanosis or extreme pallor (despite oxygen being given)

- sweating

- bradycardia.

In children, recognition of respiratory failure is based on the full assessment of respiratory effort and efficacy, and the identification of evidence of respiratory inadequacy on major organs.

Work of breathing

Evidence of increased work of breathing is based on observation of the following:

- increased respiratory rate

- intercostal recession

- sternal recession

- subcostal recession

- use of accessory muscles (e.g. nasal flaring)

- head bobbing.

Respiratory rate

Tachypnoea is frequently the first indication of respiratory insufficiency. Normal respiratory rates vary with age and this must be considered when determining the presence of tachypnoea (Table 1.1).

Changes in respiratory rate over time are very important. An increasing respiratory rate represents increasing physiological compensation to offset the deterioration in respiratory function. A sudden reduction in the respiratory rate in an acutely ill child is an ominous sign and may be a pre-terminal event. Causes may include exhaustion, central nervous system depression or hypothermia. Fatigue is always an important consideration in children: an infant with a respiratory rate of 80 min^{-1} will tire quickly.

Recession

Recession (or retractions) may be sternal, subcostal or intercostal. The degree of recession gives an indication of the severity of respiratory disorder. Infants and young children can exhibit significant recession with relatively mild to moderate respiratory compromise, owing to their highly compliant chest wall. However, in children over approximately 5 years (by which age the chest wall is less compliant) recession is a sign of significant respiratory compromise.

Use of accessory muscles

When the work of breathing is increased, the sternocleidomastoid muscles in the neck are often used as accessory respiratory muscles. In infants, this may cause the head to bob up and down with each breath. This 'head bobbing' actually reduces the efficiency of each breath.

'See-saw' respiration

A breathing pattern, described as 'see-saw' respiration, is sometimes observed in severe respiratory compromise. It is the paradoxical movement of the abdomen during inspiration (i.e. the abdomen expands and the thorax retracts as the diaphragm contracts). This is inefficient respiration because the tidal volume is reduced, despite the increased muscular effort.

Inspiratory and expiratory noises

Normally, the airway above the thoracic inlet (extrathoracic) narrows and the airway below (intrathoracic) widens during the inspiratory phase of breathing. This pattern reverses on expiration. Observing the timing of an abnormal noise can indicate the site of airway obstruction. The presence of a high-pitched inspiratory noise (stridor) is characteristic of an upper airway (extrathoracic) obstruction and is due to rapid, turbulent flow through a narrowed portion of the upper tracheal airway. In severe obstruction, the stridor may also occur on expiration (biphasic stridor) but is usually less pronounced than it is during inspiration.

Wheezing is generally an expiratory noise. It is indicative of lower (intrathoracic) airway narrowing, usually at bronchiolar level, and may be audible with the ear, or only on chest auscultation with a stethoscope.

The volume of airway noises is not indicative of the severity of respiratory compromise; diminishing noises may be indicative of increasing airway obstruction or exhaustion of the child.

Grunting

Grunting is mainly heard in neonates and small infants, but can also occur in young children. It is the result of exhaling against a partially closed glottis, and is an attempt to generate a positive end-expiratory pressure thus preventing airway collapse at the end of expiration. Grunting is generally associated with 'stiff' lungs (e.g. respiratory distress syndrome, pulmonary oedema, atelectasis). Regardless of the underlying condition, grunting is an indication of severe respiratory compromise.

Nostril flaring

Flaring of the nostrils is often seen in infants and young children with increased respiratory effort.

Position

Children in respiratory distress will usually adopt a position to maximise their respiratory capacity. In upper airway obstruction, they often adopt a 'sniffing the morning air' position to optimise their upper airway patency. In generalised or lower respiratory problems, children often sit forward, supporting their weight on their arms, and holding on to (or wrap their arms around) their knees. This position results in a degree of shoulder girdle 'splinting', which enhances accessory muscle use. The child should be supported in the position of optimal airway maximisation/comfort for them and have oxygen therapy given accordingly.

The degree of respiratory distress generally provides clinical evidence of the severity of respiratory insufficiency. However, there are three general exceptions to this (Table 2.2).

Table 2.2 Exceptions to increased work of breathing in respiratory failure

1. Exhaustion – children who have had severe respiratory compromise for some time may have progressed to decompensation and no longer show signs of increased work of breathing

   Exhaustion is a pre-terminal event

2. Neuromuscular diseases (e.g. muscular dystrophy)

3. Central respiratory depression – reduced respiratory drive results in respiratory inadequacy (e.g. encephalopathy, medications such as morphine)

Efficacy of breathing

The infant's relatively higher metabolic rate and oxygen consumption accounts for their increased respiratory rates (Table 1.1). Thus the effectiveness of breathing can be assessed by respiratory rate together with tidal volume, which in turn is evaluated by observation of chest movement, palpation, auscultation and percussion. Additional information can be easily obtained by non-invasive pulse oximetry.

Chest movement, palpation and percussion

Observation of chest movement demonstrates the extent and symmetry of chest expansion. As well as revealing increased work of breathing, observing the movement of the chest wall can help identify diminished or asymmetrical respiratory effort.

Palpation of the chest wall may identify deformities, surgical emphysema or crepitus.

Percussion of the chest wall can demonstrate areas of collapse (dullness) or hyper-resonance (e.g. in pneumothorax).

Chest auscultation

When listening with a stethoscope, air entry should be heard in all areas of the lungs. Volume of air movement occurring with inspiration and expiration can be estimated by auscultation. It is useful to compare the areas on one side of the chest with the other.

A very quiet or near silent chest indicates a dangerously reduced tidal volume and is an ominous sign.

Pulse oximetry

A pulse oximeter should be used on any child with potential respiratory failure to provide an assessment of his arterial oxygen saturation. A peripheral arterial oxygen saturation (SpO_2) of < 90% in air or < 95% in supplemental oxygen indicates respiratory failure.

It should be noted that SpO_2 measurements are unreliable when a child has a poor peripheral circulation. When SpO_2 is less than 70% pulse oximetry is inaccurate although trends will still be reliable.

Effects of respiratory inadequacy on other body organs

Ongoing respiratory compromise rapidly affects other body organs/systems.

Heart rate

Hypoxia initially causes tachycardia. As this is a non-specific sign it needs to be considered alongside other clinical signs. Severe or prolonged hypoxia ultimately leads to bradycardia and therefore it is important to observe for trends rather than absolute values in heart rate. In a severely hypoxic child, bradycardia is a pre-terminal sign.

Skin perfusion

Hypoxia produces vasoconstriction and pallor of the skin. As their clinical condition deteriorates, the child's colour may become mottled before cyanosis appears centrally (lips and mouth). Cyanosis is not a reliable indicator of the degree of hypoxia; it may never be observed in a profoundly hypoxic child if there is significant anaemia. However, in a child with acute respiratory compromise, the development of **central cyanosis is a late indication of severe hypoxia and is a pre-terminal sign.**

Conscious level

Hypoxia and/or hypercapnia initially lead to agitation and/or drowsiness. Ongoing cerebral hypoxia ultimately results in loss of consciousness. In infants and young children, initial cerebral hypoxia may be difficult to detect but their parents/carers frequently report that the baby/child is not responding to them as usual. This information is important and should not be ignored. The level of consciousness should be assessed using the AVPU score (Table 2.3).

Generalised hypotonia also accompanies cerebral hypoxia.

Table 2.3 The level of consciousness
A ALERT
V responds to VOICE
P responds to PAIN
U UNRESPONSIVE to painful stimuli

The management of respiratory compromise

The treatment of breathing problems is dependent on achieving a patent airway and effective delivery of oxygen. The method of oxygen administration will vary according to the child's clinical condition and age. Children who have adequate spontaneous breathing should have high-flow oxygen delivered in a manner that is non-threatening (when agitated the child's airflow will become turbulent and resistance to flow will increase) and best tolerated by them (e.g. from a free-flow device held by their parents, a non-rebreathe facemask or nasal cannulae).

When breathing is inadequate (or absent) high-flow oxygen should be delivered by ventilation with a bag and mask system. In situations where the child is exhausted and is likely to need ongoing respiratory support, tracheal intubation may be indicated.

During resuscitation use 100% oxygen to maximise oxygen delivery to the tissues.

When the patient is stabilised adjust the inspired oxygen concentration to maintain a SpO_2 of 94–98%. If pulse oximetry (with a reliable reading) is unavailable, continue oxygen via a reservoir mask until definitive monitoring or assessment of oxygenation is available.

C: Circulatory problems

The appropriate management of the airway and ventilation (breathing) is the priority in all seriously ill children and should be addressed before considering their circulatory status.

Circulatory failure and shock

Shock is a clinical state where the delivery of oxygenated blood (and associated delivery of nutrients e.g. glucose) to the body tissues is inadequate for metabolic demand. Additionally, the removal of cellular waste (e.g. CO_2, lactic acid) may also be impaired.

Circulatory failure refers to insufficient blood being delivered to the body's tissues.

Shock may occur with increased, normal or decreased cardiac output (CO) or blood pressure (BP). Initially, the child's body can physiologically compensate for reduced tissue perfusion. However, when blood pressure starts to fall, as seen in circulatory failure, perfusion of the vital organs (e.g. brain, myocardium, kidneys) becomes increasingly compromised.

Compensated circulatory failure may have a normal blood pressure, but signs of abnormal perfusion, tachycardia, poor skin perfusion, weak peripheral pulse, tachypnoea and reduced urine output are observed.

Decompensated circulatory failure is present when hypotension develops and vital organ perfusion is compromised. The clinical signs of inadequate tissue perfusion are much more apparent.

Aetiology of shock

Shock can arise from circulatory or respiratory failure. Most children in shock, whatever its aetiology, have some degree of cardiovascular dysfunction requiring more than one type of treatment (i.e. managing the airway, breathing and circulation).

The most common causes of circulatory failure in children are hypovolaemia, sepsis or anaphylaxis.

Hypovolaemic shock: characterised by decreased circulating volume (preload). It may result from severe fluid loss (as in dehydration) or haemorrhage.

Distributive shock: typified by inadequate distribution of blood, so that the blood flow is insufficient for the metabolic demand of the tissues (e.g. anaphylaxis, sepsis or neurogenic).

Cardiogenic shock: circulatory failure is less commonly the result of a primary cardiac problem due to congenital or acquired heart disease (e.g. cardiomyopathy, myocarditis or following cardiac surgery).

Obstructive shock: an uncommon cause of circulatory failure due to obstruction of blood flow to/from the heart (e.g. tension pneumothorax, cardiac tamponade or constrictive pericarditis).

Dissociative shock: characterised by insufficient oxygen carrying capacity of the blood (e.g. anaemia or carbon monoxide poisoning).

Recognition of circulatory failure

In children, the recognition of circulatory failure is based on a complete cardiovascular assessment, looking for the effects of any circulatory insufficiency on major organs.

Parameters evaluated include:

- heart rate
- pulse volume
- capillary refill time
- blood pressure
- end organ perfusion status.

Heart rate

The heart rate initially rises to maintain cardiac output.

Sinus tachycardia is a common response to many situations (e.g. pain, anxiety, fever) but it is also seen in hypoxia, hypercapnia and hypovolaemia. When tachycardia is accompanied by other signs of circulatory insufficiency, it is evidence of the body's attempts at physiological compensation. When the increased heart rate is unable to maintain adequate tissue perfusion, the tissue hypoxia and acidosis result in bradycardia. The presence of bradycardia is a pre-terminal sign, indicating that cardiorespiratory arrest is imminent.

Pulse volume

Feeling for the volume (or amplitude) of central pulses (e.g. femoral, carotid, brachial pulses) gives a subjective indication of stroke volume (SV); as SV decreases, so does the pulse amplitude. In progressive circulatory failure, the pulse amplitude diminishes, becomes weak and thready before finally, it is impalpable. Simultaneous palpation and comparison of central and peripheral pulses (e.g. radial and carotid) may be useful. Peripheral pulses decrease in amplitude earlier than central ones. Note that caution is required in their interpretation when vasoconstriction is present (e.g. ambient temperature is low, or in an anxious or pyrexial child).

The presence or absence of peripheral pulses is neither a specific nor sensitive indicator of circulatory compromise, but is useful in conjunction with other clinical signs. **However, diminishing central pulses are a pre-terminal sign, indicating that cardiorespiratory arrest is imminent.**

Capillary refill and skin colour

The skin of a healthy child is warm to touch unless the ambient temperature is low. Their capillary refill time (CRT) is normally < 2 s, but when there is decreased skin perfusion, the CRT is prolonged.

Evaluation of CRT is best performed by applying cutaneous pressure on the centre of the sternum for 5 s. Following removal of the pressure, the blanching of the skin should disappear within 2 s. A slower refill time (i.e. prolonged CRT) is indicative of poor skin perfusion. A pyrexial child with hypovolaemia will have a prolonged CRT, despite having a raised body temperature. A low ambient temperature or poor local lighting conditions reduces the accuracy of CRT. The CRT should be considered in context of the accompanying cardiovascular signs.

Initially, hypoxia produces vasoconstriction and hence the child appears pale. As their clinical condition deteriorates, the child's colour becomes mottled and ultimately cyanosed. Cyanosis due to circulatory failure is initially peripheral, whereas hypoxia due to respiratory failure results in central cyanosis.

Peripheral vasoconstriction and decreased perfusion may also be indicated by a demarcation line between warm and cold skin. This can be detected by running the back of your hand up the child's limb. The demarcation line will travel towards the trunk over time if the child's condition is deteriorating, and vice versa if it is improving.

Blood pressure

In most forms of shock, the BP is initially maintained within the normal range (Table 1.3) for the child as a result of the body's compensatory mechanisms (e.g. tachycardia, vasoconstriction, increased myocardial contractility). Only when compensation is no longer possible, does hypotension occur and a decompensated state results.

In hypovolaemia, **approximately 40%** of the child's total circulating volume can be lost before hypotension occurs. This means that BP only drops at a late stage in hypovolaemia (e.g. trauma, diarrhoeal illness, gut necrosis). It is therefore important that compensated circulatory failure is detected and managed at an early stage (i.e. before BP drops and decompensation occurs).

Regardless of the method used to obtain the BP (auscultatory or oscillometric) it is important that the appropriate cuff size is used. The cuff width should be > 80% of the child's upper arm length, and the bladder cover more than 40% of the circumference of their arm. The same size cuff should be used on each occasion that the BP is measured.

Hypotension is a sign of physiological decompensation and indicates imminent cardiorespiratory arrest.

Effects of circulatory inadequacy on other body organs

Ongoing circulatory compromise rapidly affects other body organs/systems:

Respiratory system

The metabolic acidosis that results from circulatory compromise leads to tachypnoea. However, there will not initially be other signs of increased work of breathing.

Conscious level

Hypoxia and/or hypercapnia initially lead to agitation and/or drowsiness. Progressive cerebral hypoxia ultimately results in loss of consciousness. In infants and young children, initial cerebral hypoxia may be difficult to detect but their parents/carers frequently report that the baby/child is not responding to them as usual and, as in respiratory failure, this information should not be ignored. The level of consciousness should be assessed by the AVPU score.

Generalised hypotonia also accompanies cerebral hypoxia.

Urine output

Information regarding the degree of reduced renal perfusion can be obtained by measuring the output of urine. A urinary output of < 2 mL kg^{-1} h^{-1} in infants or < 1 mL kg^{-1} h^{-1} in children older than 1 year, is an indication of inadequate renal perfusion. Asking parents/carers about the child's urine output (e.g. the number of wet nappies, six being the average that would be expected per day) may reveal a history of oliguria or anuria.

Management of circulatory compromise

The treatment of circulatory problems is dependent on achieving a patent airway and effectively managing ventilation with appropriate delivery of high-flow oxygen before turning attention to circulatory procedures.

Immediately life-threatening causes of circulatory failure (e.g. massive or continuing haemorrhage, tension pneumothorax) must be sought and urgently treated.

Insertion of at least one large bore vascular cannula should be performed rapidly. This can be achieved by either intravenous or intraosseous routes.

Unless contraindicated (e.g. cardiac failure) volume replacement should be started using 20 mL kg^{-1} boluses of isotonic salt solution (i.e. 0.9% saline). Glucose containing fluids with low sodium levels should NEVER be used for resuscitation, only to correct for low blood glucose levels.

The use of vasoactive medications may be needed (circulatory access procedures, fluids and medications are described in Chapter 5).

Cardiorespiratory failure

Bradycardia, hypotension, bradypnoea, gasping and apnoea are terminal events preceding imminent cardiorespiratory arrest.

If any of the following signs are present, immediate intervention should be undertaken:

- coma or alteration of consciousness
- exhaustion
- cyanosis
- tachypnoea (RR > 60 min^{-1})
- HR < 100 min^{-1} for newborn
- HR > 180 min^{-1} or < 80 min^{-1} before 1 year (note: chest compressions in all ages commenced at HR < 60 min^{-1})
- HR > 160 min^{-1} or < 60 min^{-1} after 1 year
- seizures.

A rapid assessment must be made of every child in whom respiratory, circulatory or cardiorespiratory failure is suspected.

D: Disability – central neurological assessment

Following the appropriate management of the child's airway, ventilation and circulation, their neurological status should be evaluated.

Whilst both respiratory and circulatory failure can have central neurological effects, some neurological conditions may affect the respiratory and circulatory systems.

Neurological function

Conscious level

A rapid assessment of the child's conscious level can be determined by the AVPU score (Table 2.3).

If required, the painful stimulus should be delivered either by applying pressure to the supraorbital ridge or rubbing the sternum. A child who is only responsive to painful (P) stimuli has a significant degree of neurological derangement equivalent to a Glasgow coma score of approximately 8.

Pupils

The size and reactivity of pupils can be affected by a number of things, including medications, intracranial pressure and cerebral lesions. Important signs to look for are pupil dilatation, inequality and non-reactivity of the child's pupils. These features potentially indicate serious brain dysfunction.

Posture

Seriously ill children become hypotonic and floppy. However, if there is serious brain dysfunction, stiff posturing may be demonstrated. This posturing (which may only be evident when a painful stimulus is applied) can be decorticate (flexed arms and extended legs) or decerebrate (extended arms and legs); both indicate serious brain dysfunction and may be signs of raised intracranial pressure.

Blood glucose

Bed-side blood glucose estimation should be performed in all seriously ill children. The increased metabolic rate associated with acute illness leads to increased use of glucose. Infants and small children do not have large glycogen liver stores which can be broken down to generate more glucose and therefore may become hypoglycaemic with any acute illness particularly when oral intake is reduced.

Effects on other systems of central neurological failure

Central neurological dysfunction may affect other body systems.

Respiratory system

Comatose children with brain dysfunction may exhibit abnormal respiratory patterns (e.g. hyperventilation, Cheyne-Stoke respiratory pattern (alternate periods of hyperventilation and apnoea) or complete apnoea).

Circulatory system

Raised intracranial pressure causes the Cushing's triad (abnormal breathing pattern with bradycardia and hypertension). This is a late and pre-terminal sign of neurological failure.

E: Exposure

To ensure that no additional significant clinical information (e.g. rashes) is missed, examine the child fully by exposing their body. Appropriate measures to minimise heat loss (especially in infants) and respect dignity must be adopted at all times.

The ABCDE approach

In all seriously ill or injured children, the underlying principles of assessment, initial management and ongoing reassessments are the same. They are based on the systematic ABCDE approach (Table 2.4):

A	**Airway**
B	**Breathing**
C	**Circulation**
D	**Disability (mental status)**
E	**Exposure**

General principles of the ABCDE approach

- Ensure personal safety.

- Observe the child generally to determine the overall level of illness (i.e. do they look seriously unwell; are they interacting with parents/care givers).

- Speak to the child and assess the appropriateness of their response; ask the parents about the child's 'usual' behaviour.

- If they are unconscious and unresponsive to your voice, administer tactile stimulation. If they respond by speaking or crying, this indicates that they have a patent airway, are breathing and have cerebral perfusion. Regardless of the child's response to initial stimulation, you should move on to full assessment of ABCDE.

- Appropriate high-flow oxygen delivery should be commenced immediately.

- Vital sign monitoring should be requested early (ECG, SpO_2 and non-invasive BP monitoring).

- Circulatory access should be achieved as soon as possible. Blood test investigations and a bedside glucose estimation should be obtained.

Summary learning

- **Early recognition of the seriously ill child prevents the majority of cardiorespiratory arrests, thus reducing morbidity and mortality.**

- **The structured ABCDE approach helps ensure that potentially life-threatening problems are identified and dealt with in order of priority.**

My key take-home messages from this chapter

Table 2.4 Specific assessments and actions in initial ABCDE approach

Assessment	Information sought	Possible resultant actions
On approaching the child	**Note:** • **General appearance** • **Interaction with parent/caregiver**	
A Airway patency	Is the airway: • Patent (i.e. conscious, vocalising) • At risk • Obstructed	• Suction if indicated • Head positioning • Oropharyngeal airway • Reassess • Summon expert help
B Breathing adequacy	Note/observe/perform: • Conscious level • Air movement (look, listen, feel) • Respiratory rate • Chest expansion • Use of accessory muscles/recessions • Palpation • Percussion • Auscultation • SpO_2 and FiO_2	• Administer high-flow oxygen appropriately • Support breathing with bag-mask ventilation (BMV) as necessary • Reassess • Summon expert help
C Circulation adequacy	Note/observe/perform: • Evidence of haemorrhage/fluid loss • Conscious level • Heart rate • Capillary refill time • Presence of distal/central pulses • Pulse volume features • Skin temperature and colour • Blood pressure • Urine output	• Control any external bleeding • Attach monitoring (as appropriate to setting) • Obtain circulatory access (IV or IO) • Estimate weight • Blood samples for laboratory testing and bedside glucose estimation • Fluid bolus (10–20 mL kg^{-1}) • Reassess • Summon expert help
D Disability (conscious level)	Note: • AVPU score • Interaction with parent and surroundings • Posture and muscle tone • Pupil size and reactivity	• Reconsider A, B and C management as conscious level dictates • Establish bedside glucose estimation • Establish if any medications have been given/possibly ingested • Reassess • Summon expert help
E Exposure	Note/observe: • Evidence of any blood loss/skin lesions/wounds/drains/rashes etc • Core temperature	• Reconsider specific management e.g. antibiotics in sepsis • Consider appropriate temperature control measures • Reassess • Summon expert help

pILS

Basic Life Support

Contents

- Age definitions
- Infant and child basic life support sequence
- Recognition and management of choking
- Recovery positions

Learning outcomes

To enable you to:

- **Understand the importance of early effective basic life support (BLS) for decreasing mortality and morbidity**
- **Know how and when to activate the Emergency Medical Service (EMS) or the in-hospital clinical emergency team**
- **Explain the rationale for the sequence of steps in BLS**
- **Appreciate the importance of early appropriate choking management**
- **Understand the rationale for the different techniques of BLS employed in infants and children**

Age definitions

For the purposes of basic life support (BLS), an infant is a baby < 1 year and a child is aged between 1 year and puberty. It is neither appropriate nor necessary to formally establish the onset of puberty; if the rescuer thinks the victim is a child, they should use the paediatric guidelines.

Introduction

BLS is the combination of manoeuvres and skills that, without the use of technical adjuncts, provides recognition and management of a child in cardiac or respiratory arrest and 'buys time' until he can receive more advanced treatment.

BLS must be started as rapidly as possible. Its main objective is to achieve sufficient oxygenation to 'protect' the brain and other vital organs. Ideally, everyone should possess BLS knowledge and skills. The sequence of actions in BLS is known as cardiopulmonary resuscitation (CPR). BLS is more effective when the rescuer is proficient in its delivery, but even suboptimal CPR gives a better result than no CPR at all. Hence rescuers unable or unwilling to provide mouth-to-mouth ventilation should be encouraged to perform at least compression-only CPR.

BLS can be undertaken without any adjuncts; however expired air ventilation provides only 16–17% oxygen, therefore oxygen should be given as soon as possible. The trained healthcare provider must provide bag-mask ventilation (BMV) with oxygen as soon as the necessary equipment is available.

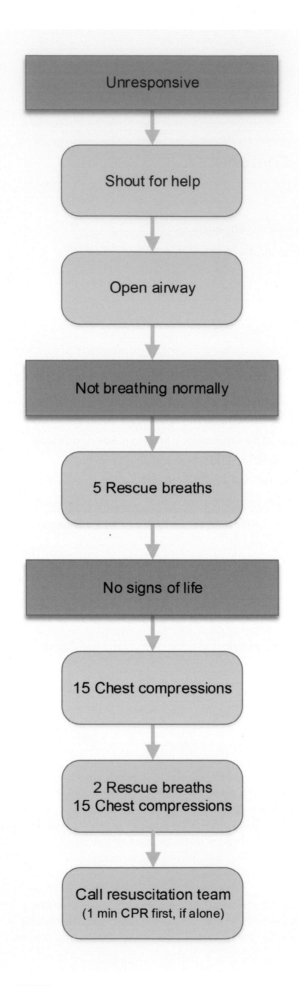

Figure 3.1 Paediatric BLS algorithm G2015

Background

In the management of the collapsed child, a number of factors affect the chances of a good outcome. The most important is the early recognition and appropriate intervention in children who exhibit signs of respiratory and/or circulatory compromise. Prevention of cardiorespiratory arrest by the optimal management of respiratory distress and/or circulatory failure will improve the prognosis (Chapters 1 and 2).

There will always be some children in whom respiratory and/or circulatory collapse cannot be prevented. For these children, early BLS, rapid activation of the Emergency Medical Service (EMS) or in-hospital clinical emergency team, and prompt, effective advanced life support are crucial in improving mortality and morbidity.

BLS sequence

The single lay rescuer should follow the adult sequence for children except that they should (ideally) attempt 5 initial rescue breaths and perform 1 min of CPR before going for help.

The BLS algorithm (Figure 3.1) and sequence described below is for **healthcare providers** who may occasionally start BLS alone but would normally work in a team.

Although unusual, primary cardiac arrest in ventricular fibrillation (VF) or pulseless ventricular tachycardia (pVT) does occasionally occur in children. If this situation is likely, such as with the sudden, witnessed collapse of a child with a known cardiac condition, optimal outcome will depend on early defibrillation. In this situation a lone rescuer should activate the EMS <u>before</u> starting BLS and use an automated external defibrillator (AED), if available.

However, for the majority of children who suffer cardiorespiratory arrest, the recommended sequence of events is based on two facts:

1. Cardiorespiratory arrest is hypoxic in origin and therefore the priority is prompt oxygenation (provided by rescue breaths).

2. The most common cardiac arrhythmia is profound bradycardia deteriorating into asystole; hence effective BLS is more important than access to a defibrillator.

Rescuers should follow the specific order of steps in BLS because if one manoeuvre is missed or incorrectly performed, the effectiveness of the next step is likely to also be compromised (Figure 3.2).

S – Safety

Quickly assess the situation and ensure the safety of first, the rescuer(s) and then that of the child; although the potential hazards may be different, this is equally important whether the situation occurs within or outside the healthcare environment.

S	**Safety**
S	**Stimulate**
S	**Shout for assistance**
A	**Airway**
B	**Breathing**
C	**Circulation**
R	**Reassess**

Figure 3.2 BLS sequence

All bodily fluids should be treated as potentially infectious; put on gloves as soon as practicable and use barrier devices for ventilation (e.g. pocket mask) if available. Whilst the efficacy of face shields is uncertain and they may not reliably prevent transmission of infection, their use affords some protection and may make it more acceptable for the receipt or delivery of rescue breaths.

On approaching the child, and before touching them, look for any clues as to what may have caused the emergency as this may influence the way the child is managed (e.g. any suspicion of head or neck injury necessitates consideration of cervical spine immobilisation).

S – Stimulate

It is important to establish the responsiveness of the apparently unconscious child by tactile and verbal stimulation as they may not be in a critical condition. This can be done by stabilising the child's head, placing one hand on their forehead and then tugging their hair, whilst calling their name or telling them to "wake up". A child should never be shaken vigorously.

If the child responds (e.g. moves, cries or talks), his clinical status and any further potential dangers should be assessed, and if necessary, help obtained.

If there is no response continue with BLS as described below.

S – Shout

If there is only one rescuer, they must not leave the child (or delay BLS to use a mobile telephone), but shout for "help" as they start BLS. If there is another person present, that individual should be asked to summon the EMS.

This second rescuer should get help by dialling either 999 or 112 for EMS out of hospital, or 2222 for the hospital clinical emergency team. They must be able to convey the specific information listed in Table 3.1.

Table 3.1 Information required when requesting EMS	
National 999 or 112 ambulance request	**In-hospital 2222 request**
Precise location of the emergency	Precise location of the emergency
Type of emergency (e.g. infant in cardiorespiratory arrest, child in road traffic accident)	Specific clinical emergency team required (e.g. paediatric, paediatric trauma)
Number and age of victim(s)	Any other local policy requirements
Severity and urgency of the situation	

The caller should only end the phone call once the operator confirms no further information is needed. They should then return to the rescuer(s) delivering BLS and inform them that the EMS has been activated. If the event is within a healthcare environment, appropriate clinical emergency equipment should also be taken to the bedside.

A – Airway

In the unconscious child, the tongue is likely to at least partly occlude the airway. This can usually be overcome by using a head tilt and chin lift manoeuvre or, if necessary, by performing a jaw thrust.

Head tilt and chin lift

The head tilt is a simple and effective initial manoeuvre. To perform the head tilt, approach the child from the side, place one hand on their forehead and gently tilt their head back. In infants, the head should be placed in a neutral position (Figure 3.3). For the child, a 'sniffing' position that causes some extension of the head on the neck will be required (Figure 3.4).

The chin lift is performed by placing the fingertips of the rescuer's other hand on the bony part of the child's lower jaw, and lifting the chin upwards. It is essential that the rescuer takes care not to compress the soft tissues under the child's jaw as this will occlude the airway.

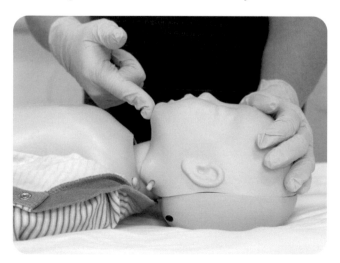

Figure 3.3 Head tilt and chin lift in an infant (neutral position)

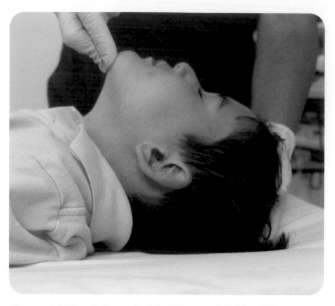

Figure 3.4 Head tilt and chin lift in a child ('sniffing position)

Jaw thrust

This is the preferred airway opening manoeuvre when cervical spine immobilisation is required. To perform a jaw thrust, the rescuer should approach the child from behind and place their hands on either side of the child's head. Two or three fingertips of both hands should be placed under both angles of the child's lower jaw. With their thumbs resting gently on the child's cheeks, the rescuer should then lift the jaw upwards (Figure 3.5).

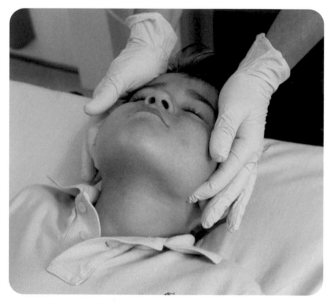

Figure 3.5 Jaw thrust manoeuvre in a child

Whichever method of airway opening is used, it is also important for rescuers to look in the child's mouth to ensure there is no obvious foreign body present. If a foreign body is seen and the rescuer is confident that they can remove it with a single finger sweep, this can be attempted; however, blind finger sweeps should never be performed. The management of choking is discussed later in this chapter.

B – Breathing

Assessing for normal breathing

After opening the airway, the rescuer needs to assess the child for effective, normal breathing. The best way to do this is to 'look, listen and feel' whilst maintaining the airway opening manoeuvre.

LOOK	**for chest (and abdominal) movements**
LISTEN	**for airflow at the mouth and nose (+/- additional noises)**
FEEL	**for airflow at the mouth and nose**

The rescuer positions themselves with a cheek just a few centimetres above the child's mouth and nose, and looks along the child's chest **for no more than 10 seconds** (Figures 3.6 and 3.7).

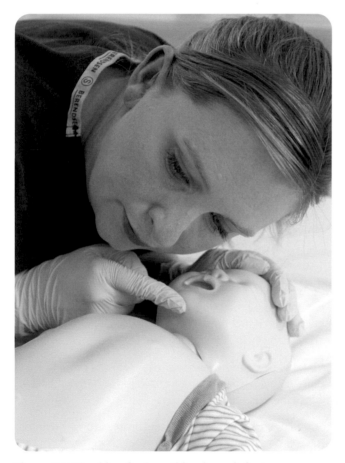

Figure 3.6 Checking for breathing in an infant

If the child is breathing normally and effectively, the rescuer should maintain the airway opening manoeuvre whilst help is summoned; however, if there is no-one else to activate the EMS, the rescuer must do this themselves.

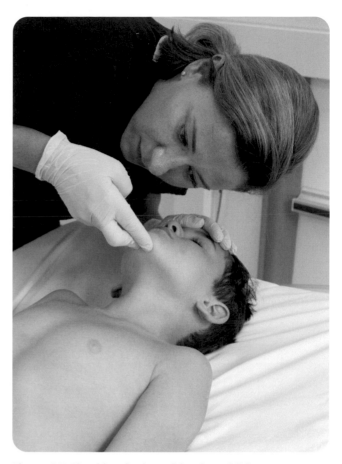

Figure 3.7 Checking for breathing in a child

Unless contraindicated (i.e. suspicion of spinal injury) the child should be placed in a safe position lying on their side (described later in this chapter) until further help arrives.

If the child is not breathing normally, or they are simply gasping ineffectively (agonal breathing), the rescuer must attempt five rescue breaths. Agonal breathing is infrequent or irregular, noisy gasps, which must not be confused with normal breathing.

Delivery of expired air rescue breaths

The aim of rescue breaths is to deliver oxygen to the child's lungs. Until an appropriate ventilation device is available, expired air rescue breathing is required. The effectiveness of rescue breaths is assessed by observing the rise and fall of the child's chest wall; rescuers may need to adapt the pressure and volume of breath delivery to the individual child to ensure that chest movement is obtained with each breath delivered.

Five initial rescue breaths should be attempted. Each breath should be delivered slowly (over approximately 1 s). This maximises the amount of oxygen delivered to the child's lungs and minimises the risk of gastric distension. By inhaling deeply themselves between each rescue breath, the rescuer can optimise the oxygen and minimise the carbon dioxide levels they deliver to the child. The effectiveness of the rescue breaths can only be determined by observing the rise and fall of the chest.

If chest movement is not observed with attempted delivery of a rescue breath, the rescuer must reassess the child's airway (i.e. reposition the child's head) and ensure they have an adequate seal between their mouth and the child's face before they attempt the next breath. If, despite repositioning the child's head and having an adequate seal, the rescuer is still unable to achieve movement of the child's chest after five attempts, the likelihood of choking should be considered and the rescuer should move straight to chest compressions.

Mouth-to-mouth and nose rescue breathing

This is the recommended technique for giving expired air rescue breaths to an infant. The rescuer places their mouth around both the mouth and nose to create a tight seal, and then blows into the infant (Figure 3.8). If it is not possible to cover both the mouth and nose, the rescuer can choose to blow into either the infant's mouth or nose (with the nostrils occluded or the mouth closed, to minimise escape of air).

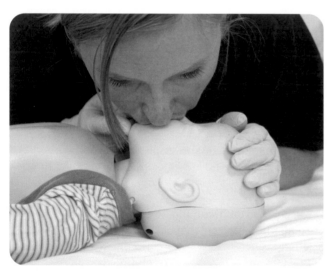

Figure 3.8 Mouth-to-mouth and nose rescue breath delivery in an infant

Mouth-to-mouth rescue breathing

This is the recommended technique for giving expired air rescue breaths to a child (Figure 3.9). The rescuer places their mouth over the child's mouth, creating a seal. Using the fingers of their hand at the top of the child's head, the rescuer occludes the child's nostrils to ensure that the rescue breath does not escape through the child's nose.

C – Circulation

Assessing for 'signs of life'

After the five initial rescue breaths attempts are given, the rescuer needs to determine whether the child has an adequate spontaneous circulation, or if they also require chest compressions. The time taken for any rescuer to assess the circulation should **not exceed 10 s.** Observe the child for signs of life.

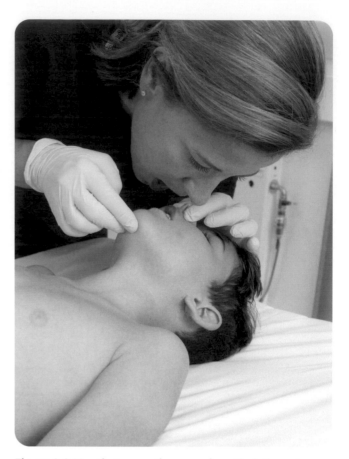

Figure 3.9 Mouth-to-mouth rescue breath delivery in a child

Signs of life include:

> • **swallowing**
>
> • **vocalising**
>
> • **coughing**
>
> • **normal (not agonal) breathing**

For healthcare professionals who are trained in pulse checking, a central pulse can be palpated, whilst simultaneously looking for 'signs of life'.

In infants the recommended sites for central pulse palpation are the femoral or brachial artery (Figure 3.10). In the child it is the femoral or carotid artery (Figure 3.11).

If there are no 'signs of life', chest compressions should be started immediately, unless the rescuer is **certain** they can feel a definite pulse > 60 min[-1] within 10 s. If there is any doubt, start chest compressions.

If there are 'signs of life' and/or a pulse is found (i.e. > 60 min[-1]), the rescuer should reassess the child's breathing. If breathing is absent or inadequate (e.g. agonal breathing) then rescue breathing should be continued at a rate of 12–20 breaths min[-1].

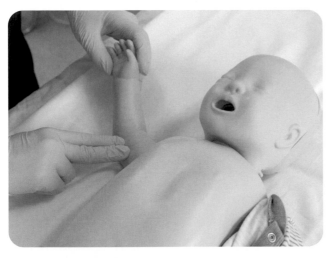

Figure 3.10 Brachial pulse palpation on an infant

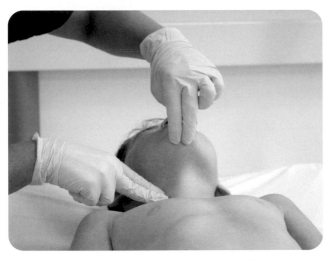

Figure 3.11 Carotid pulse palpation on a child

The child's breathing and circulation should be frequently reassessed and BLS continued until either the EMS arrives to take over, or until the child starts to breathe spontaneously.

If effective spontaneous breathing is established, and there is no suspicion of cervical spine trauma, the child should be placed in a safe position lying on their side.

Principles of chest compressions

Chest compressions are serial, rhythmic compressions of the anterior chest wall, intended to cause blood to flow to vital organ tissues in an attempt to keep them viable until return of spontaneous circulation (ROSC) is achieved.

The recommended ratio of chest compressions to ventilations for infants and children is 15:2. However, a lone healthcare professional may choose to use the standard adult ratio of 30:2 to avoid changing frequently between rescue breathing and chest compressions. For simplicity, lay persons are taught to use the adult 30:2 ratio. Whichever ratio is used, chest compressions must be performed effectively and to a high quality to achieve the best outcomes.

The rate of chest compressions should be 100–120 min⁻¹; it should be noted that when interspersed with rescue breaths, the actual number of compressions delivered will be less than this.

The rate of chest compressions should be $100–120\ min^{-1}$; it should be noted that when interspersed with rescue breaths, the actual number of compressions delivered will be less than this.

Effective chest compression is facilitated by ensuring the child or infant is lying on a firm flat surface. It requires depression of the infant's chest by approximately 4 cm and the child's chest by approximately 5 cm with equal time spent in the compression and relaxation phases.

During the relaxation phase of each compression, the rescuer should release the pressure whilst leaving their hand(s)/fingers in position on the child's chest wall.

At the end of each series of chest compressions, the hand(s) /fingers must be removed from the child's chest in order to effectively perform airway opening manoeuvres and give two rescue breaths.

Landmarking for chest compressions

In all infants and children, deliver chest compressions over the lower half of the sternum. In order to avoid compressing the upper abdomen, locate the xiphisternum at the angle where the lower costal margins meet and compress one finger's breadth above this point (Figure 3.12).

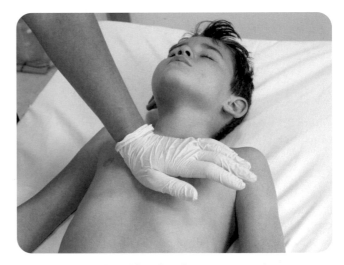

Figure 3.12 Landmarking for chest compressions on a child

Performing chest compressions

Infant chest compression

Two-finger technique

This is the recommended method of infant chest compression for the lone rescuer. Having landmarked as described above, place two fingers of one hand in the correct position on the sternum and depress it by 4 cm (at least one third of the anteroposterior diameter) (Figure 3.13 and Figure 3.14).

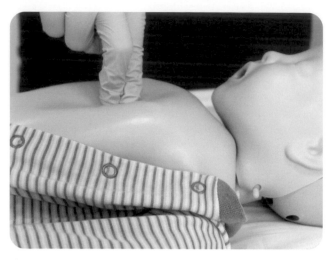

Figure 3.13 Two-finger chest compression on an infant – depression phase

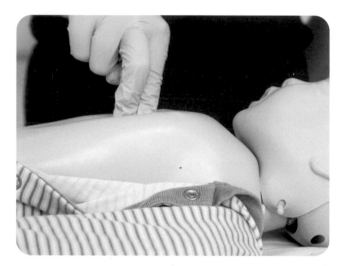

Figure 3.14 Two-finger chest compression on an infant – relaxation phase

Two-thumb encircling technique

This is the recommended method of infant chest compression for two rescuers. There is evidence that this method delivers greater cardiac output than the two-finger technique, but it is a difficult technique for a single rescuer to perform in a timely and effective manner. It is therefore usually reserved for in-hospital resuscitation where there are two rescuers and ventilation delivery devices can be used.

The two-thumb encircling technique requires a healthcare professional to be positioned at the infant's head to maintain the airway and deliver ventilation. A second rescuer, at the infant's side (or at their feet), places their two thumbs side-by-side in the correct position on the lower half of the sternum (Figure 3.15). In a very small baby, the thumbs may be placed one on top of the other. The rest of the rescuer's hands are then able to support the infant's back as they encircle the chest wall. Chest compressions are delivered as described previously, it is very important to allow full chest recoil with this method.

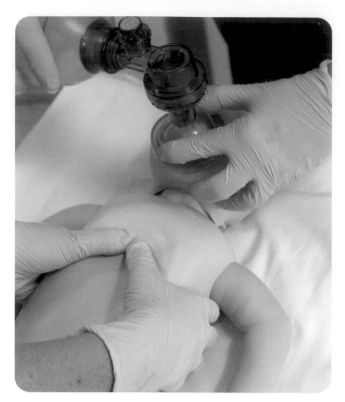

Figure 3.15 Two-thumb encircling chest compressions on an infant

Child chest compression

Having confirmed landmarks as previously described, the rescuer should position themselves at one side of the child, and place the heel of one hand along the long axis of the lower half of the child's sternum. The fingers should be raised off the chest so that pressure is exerted only through the heel of the hand and on to the sternum.

By positioning themselves so that their elbow is locked straight, and their shoulders are directly over the heel of their hand on the child's chest, the rescuer can use their body weight to depress the sternum by 5 cm (at least one third of the anteroposterior diameter). In larger children or for small rescuers, this is achieved more effectively by using both hands with the fingers interlocked together off the chest wall. (Figure 3.16).

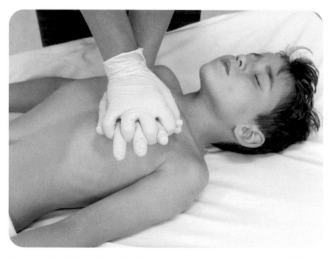

Figure 3.16 Two-handed chest compression on a child

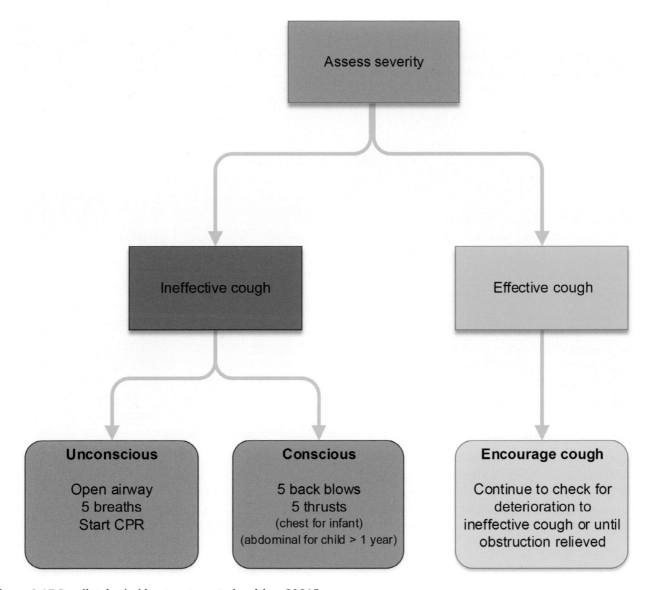

Figure 3.17 Paediatric choking treatment algorithm G2015

R – Reassess

After approximately one minute of BLS, a single rescuer should stop to go and call the EMS unless a second person was available to do this. A mobile phone may be used if available. Otherwise, if the victim is an infant or a very small child, the rescuer may be able to carry him safely to activate a telephone to summon further assistance, and then continue CPR. If the child is too large to carry, the child should be briefly left in order to activate the EMS, and BLS recommenced as soon as possible on return to the child.

If the EMS has already been activated, the rescuer should immediately resume BLS unless there are obvious 'signs of life'.

Continuation of BLS

BLS should only be stopped when:

- the child exhibits adequate 'signs of life'

- further rescuers take over resuscitation

- the single rescuer is too exhausted to continue.

As soon as the EMS and/or appropriate paediatric resuscitation equipment becomes available, advanced life support techniques can start.

Choking

When a foreign body enters their airway, a child will react immediately by coughing in an attempt to expel it. A child who is choking on a foreign body but is still able to cough effectively must be actively encouraged to do so. A spontaneous cough is not only safer, it is also probably more effective than any manoeuvre a rescuer might perform.

If coughing is absent or becoming ineffective, the child's airway is at risk of complete obstruction, which will rapidly result in asphyxiation. Any child who is unable to effectively cough as a result of foreign body aspiration, requires immediate interventions (Figure 3.17).

Recognition of choking

Choking is characterised by the sudden onset of respiratory distress associated with coughing, gagging or stridor.

The majority of choking events in infants and children occur during play or feeding, and are therefore frequently witnessed by an adult which means interventions can start immediately. However, it is important to be aware that the signs of choking (Table 3.2) can be confused with those of other causes of airway obstruction (e.g. laryngitis or epiglottitis) which require different management.

Table 3.2 Signs of choking	
General signs	
Witnessed episode	
Coughing or choking	
Sudden onset	
Recent history of playing with, or eating small objects	
Ineffective cough	**Effective cough**
Unable to vocalise	Crying or verbal response to questions
Quiet or silent cough	Loud cough
Unable to breathe	Able to take a breath before coughing
Cyanosis	
Decreasing level of consciousness	Fully responsive

Management of choking

As with BLS, quickly assess the situation and ensure the safety of the rescuer(s) and then that of the child. Although the potential hazards are different, this is equally important whether the situation occurs within or outside of the healthcare environment.

If the child is coughing effectively, no external manoeuvre is necessary. The rescuer should encourage the child's coughing and observe them closely.

If the child's coughing is absent or becoming ineffective, the rescuer must shout for help and quickly determine the child's conscious level.

Conscious infants and children

If the child is conscious but their coughing is absent or ineffective, the rescuer must deliver back blows. These are intended to loosen the object in order for the child to be able to then expel it. If back blows do not relieve the airway obstruction, thrusts should be given; chest thrusts for infants and abdominal thrusts for children. These thrusts are intended as an 'artificial cough'; they increase the intrathoracic pressure which will facilitate expulsion of the foreign body.

Delivery of back blows to an infant

1. To deliver back blows safely, the rescuer should either sit on a chair or kneel on the floor and hold the infant in a head downwards, prone position across their lap Figure 3.18.

2. The rescuer must support the infant's head by placing the thumb of one hand at the angle of the lower jaw, and one or two fingers from the same hand at the

same point on the other side of the infant's face. Care must be taken not to compress the soft tissues under the infant's jaw.

3. Up to 5 sharp back blows should be delivered to the middle of the infant's back, between their scapulae, with the heel of the rescuer's other hand.

The aim is to relieve the obstruction with each individual back blow rather than to give all five.

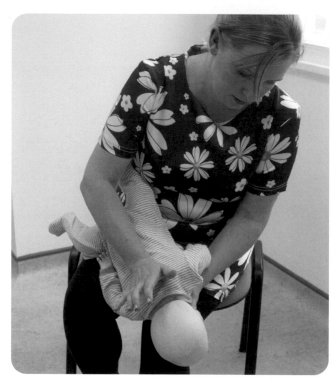

Figure 3.18 Delivery of back blows to an infant

Delivery of back blows to a child

1. To maximise effectiveness, the rescuer should try to support the child in a head downwards position (Figure 3.19). If the child is too large to do this safely, they should be supported in a forward-leaning position, with the rescuer delivering the back blows from behind.

2. Up to five sharp back blows should be delivered to the middle of the child's back, between their scapulae, with the heel of the rescuer's other hand.

The aim is to relieve the obstruction with each individual back blow rather than to give all five.

If back blows fail to dislodge the foreign body and the infant/child is still conscious, the rescuer should deliver thrusts. In infants these are delivered to the chest, and are similar to chest compressions. However, in children over one year, abdominal thrusts may be performed. If the clinical judgement of the rescuer is that the child is too small to tolerate abdominal thrusts, then chest thrusts can be delivered instead. **Abdominal thrusts (Heimlich manoeuvre) must not be performed on infants.**

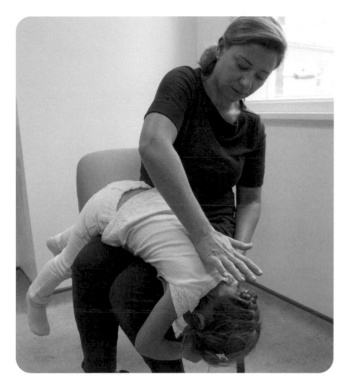

Figure 3.19 Delivery of back blows to a child

Delivery of chest thrusts to an infant

1. The rescuer should turn the infant from the head downwards, prone position they were in for back blow delivery, into a head downwards, supine position. This can be safely achieved by placement of the rescuer's free arm along the infant's back, with the hand encircling the infant's occiput. The infant should then be turned over whilst keeping their head lower than their trunk.

2. The rescuer must support the infant down their arm which is supported down (or across) their thigh.

3. The landmark for chest compressions should be identified on the infant's sternum and up to five sharp downward thrusts delivered. These thrusts are similar to chest compressions but they are sharper in nature and delivered at a slower rate.

The aim is to relieve the obstruction with each individual chest thrust rather than to give all five.

Delivery of abdominal thrusts to a child over one year

1. To maximise safety, the rescuer should stand behind the child, and support them in a forward leaning position by placing their arms underneath the child's and encircling their torso.

2. The rescuer should clench one of their fists and place it against the child's abdomen, approximately midway between the umbilicus and the xiphisternum.

3. By grasping their fist with their free hand, the rescuer should deliver the abdominal thrusts by pulling sharply

inwards and upwards up to five times (Figure 3.20). Care should be taken not to exert pressure over the xiphoid process or the lower rib cage as this may result in thoracic or intra-abdominal trauma.

The aim is to relieve the obstruction with each individual abdominal thrust rather than to give all five.

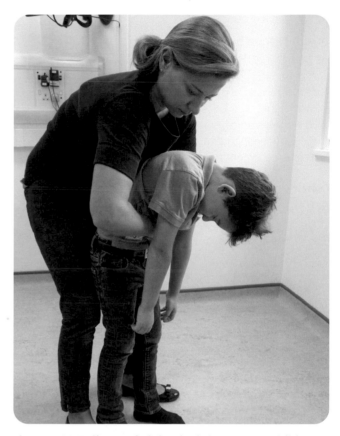

Figure 3.20 Delivery of abdominal thrusts to a child

Reassessment

Following delivery of the chest or abdominal thrusts, the rescuer must reassess the child.

If the foreign body has been successfully expelled, the child may still need medical assistance; a piece of the object may remain in the respiratory tract and cause further complications. As abdominal thrusts can cause injury, a child who has received them should be examined by a medical practitioner.

If the foreign body has not been expelled and the child remains conscious, repeat the sequence of back blows and thrusts as indicated. Do not leave the child at this stage, but call out again to ensure that the EMS has been called.

Unresponsive infants and children

If the child is, or becomes, unconscious from choking, they should be placed supine on a firm, flat surface, whilst the rescuer shouts for help. If a second rescuer is available, they should be sent to activate the EMS. If there is only one rescuer, they must not leave the child at this stage, but proceed with BLS as described earlier in this chapter, with particular attention to the following points:

Checking the mouth

Each time the airway is opened for rescue breaths, the rescuer should look to see if they can detect the foreign body in the child's mouth. If it is visible, a single finger sweep can be attempted to remove the object. However, blind or repeated finger sweeps must not be performed as these are likely to impact the object further down the pharynx and/or cause trauma.

Initial rescue breaths

When a rescue breath attempt does not result in chest wall expansion, the child's head should be repositioned before attempting the next breath. If, despite repositioning, all five rescue breaths are ineffective and the child remains unresponsive (no 'signs of life'), the rescuer should proceed straight to chest compressions without further assessment of the circulation.

Continued BLS

Continue with BLS for approximately 1 min, or 5 cycles of 15 compressions to 2 ventilations before summoning the EMS (if this has not already been done by someone else).

If the child displays signs of life, the rescuer should assess their ABC and continue as appropriate.

Recovery positions

Unless contraindicated, the unresponsive child who has effective spontaneous breathing should be placed in a safe position lying on their side (Figure 3.21).

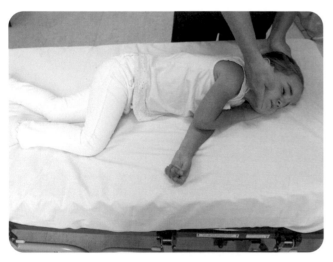

Figure 3.21 An unresponsive child in a safe side-lying position

The purpose of placing an unresponsive child in such a position is to ensure that their tongue does not fall backwards occluding their pharynx, and to reduce the potential risk of aspiration should they vomit.

There is no universally accepted 'recovery' position for children, but there are general principles to be considered when placing the child in a safe position. These include ensuring that the child:

- has a patent airway

- can drain secretions/vomit freely from their mouth

- is in a stable position that they cannot easily roll over from (this may require the placement of a rolled-up towel or blanket behind their back in small infants)

- can be easily observed

- can be easily turned on to their back if they require resuscitation interventions

- is in as near a true lateral position as possible

- has no pressure on their chest that may impede breathing.

If the child needs to be in this position for longer than one hour, they should be turned on to their other side to relieve the pressure on the lower arm.

Summary learning

- **Rescuers must always ensure their own safety before undertaking BLS.**

- **The preferred ratio of chest compressions: ventilations is 15:2 when BLS is being delivered by healthcare professionals but in some instances it may be appropriate to adopt the standard adult 30:2 sequence.**

- **One full minute of BLS should be performed by lone rescuers before they activate EMS (except on the rare occasion that a primary cardiac arrest is suspected).**

- **Management of conscious choking infants consists of back blows followed by chest thrusts.**

- **Management of conscious choking children consists of back blows followed by abdominal thrusts.**

- **Management of unconscious infants and children with choking requires BLS to be performed.**

My key take-home messages from this chapter

pILS

pILS

Management of airway and ventilation

Contents

- Airway management using positioning and adjuncts
- Oxygen delivery devices
- Assisted ventilation methods

Learning outcomes

To enable you to:
- **Understand the causes and management of airway obstruction**
- **Describe basic techniques to optimise the airway in initial resuscitation**
- **Use simple adjuncts to assist in maintaining airway patency**
- **Use simple devices for ventilation of the lungs**

Causes of upper obstruction

Airway obstruction is a common occurrence in paediatric resuscitation. It may be the primary cause of the cardiorespiratory arrest (e.g. choking) or a consequence of the underlying disease process (i.e. hypoxia), which leads to loss of consciousness. In unconscious children, the tongue can fall backwards and occlude the airway (Figure 4.1). Regardless of the cause, airway obstruction must be rapidly recognised and managed to prevent secondary hypoxic damage to the vital organs.

Recognition of airway obstruction

In a conscious child, airway obstruction may be demonstrated by difficulty in breathing and/or increased respiratory effort. In both conscious and unconscious children, there may be additional respiratory noises if the obstruction is partial, whereas respiration will be silent if there is complete obstruction.

The most effective way to detect potential airway obstruction in all children is to look, listen and feel.

LOOK	**for chest (and abdominal) movements**
LISTEN	**for airflow at the mouth and nose (+/- additional noises)**
FEEL	**for airflow at the mouth and nose**

LOOKING for breathing – during normal breathing, the chest wall expands and the abdomen is pushed slightly outwards as the diaphragm contracts. When the airway is obstructed however, the abdomen protrudes markedly and the chest is drawn inwards when the diaphragm contracts during inspiration ('see-saw' respiration). Additionally, accessory muscle usage and recession are likely to be observed. It can be difficult to differentiate these paradoxical movements from normal breathing, and you must also listen for the presence or absence of breath sounds and feel for air movement. If a clear facemask is being used, misting of the mask may be observed.

LISTENING for breathing – normal respiration is quiet. Partially obstructed breathing is noisy, whilst completely obstructed breathing will be silent.

FEELING for breathing – the movement of air on inspiration and expiration can be felt at the mouth and nose (or tracheostomy) during normal breathing. If there is airway obstruction this will be limited or absent.

Partial airway obstruction can quickly deteriorate to complete obstruction and therefore must always be considered as a potential emergency. Airway obstruction that is complete will lead to profound hypoxia, vital organ failure and cardiorespiratory arrest if the obstruction is not relieved very rapidly. Immediate action must be taken to relieve the obstruction and/or optimise the airway.

Basic techniques to optimise the airway

Conscious children

If the child is making adequate spontaneous respiratory effort, they should be supported in a position of comfort (preferably the one they naturally assume to optimise their airway). High-flow oxygen should be administered in a manner that the child will tolerate, whilst experienced help is sought.

Unconscious children

Whether or not the child is making spontaneous respiratory effort, their airway needs to be optimised immediately. This initially means positioning their head by performing either a head tilt and chin lift, or a jaw thrust manoeuvre.

Additionally, suction may be required to clear secretions, vomitus or blood.

Head positioning

By performing a head tilt and chin lift (Figure 4.2) or jaw thrust manoeuvre (Chapter 3) the rescuer can maximise the child's airway. It is important to ensure that head positioning techniques are carried out properly so that neither hyperextension (Figure 4.3) nor excessive flexion of the neck occurs, as both will make obstruction worse. The rescuer must also take care not to compress the soft tissues under the child's jaw as this can also occlude the airway.

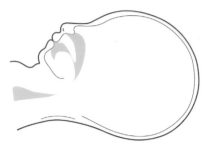

Figure 4.1 Unconscious child, the tongue falls backwards and obstructs the airway

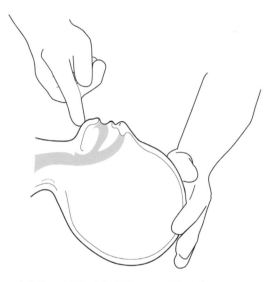

Figure 4.2 Head tilt chin lift opens the airway

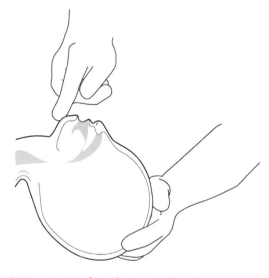

Figure 4.3 Hyperextension obstructs the airway

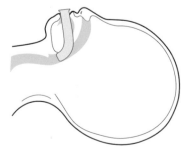

Figure 4.4 Airway adjunct keeps the tongue forward

Suction

Standard suction devices in hospital are pipeline units. They consist of a wall terminal outlet, vacuum pressure regulator, a reservoir, tubing and connector for an appropriate suction catheter to be attached.

In some low dependency hospital areas, during transportation and non-hospital environments such as GP surgeries, it is likely that the suction device available will be a portable device that is operated by battery or a hand/foot pump.

Large bore rigid suction catheters (e.g. Yankauer) are particularly useful for clearance of thick or excessive secretions and vomitus. Soft, flexible catheters in a range of sizes should also be available, these are less traumatic to use and therefore may be preferable in small children and infants. They are particularly useful for nasal suction and can also be passed through nasopharyngeal or oropharyngeal airways. However, they may not allow adequate clearance of thick or copious secretions.

Whichever catheter types are used, they should ideally have a side hole that can be occluded by the rescuer's finger to allow more control over the suction pressure generated.

Airway suction must be carried out cautiously if the child has an intact gag reflex as it may induce vomiting which can lead to aspiration.

Airway opening adjuncts

Oropharyngeal airways

The oropharyngeal airway (e.g. Guedel) is a rigid curved tube that is designed to open a channel between the base of the tongue and the posterior pharyngeal wall (Figure 4.4). They are made of plastic and are reinforced and flanged at the outer end. Available sizes range from 000 for premature infants to 4–5 for large adults (Figure 4.5).

The correctly sized airway is one that, when laid against the side of the face, has a length equal to the distance between the level of the child's incisors (or where they will be) to the angle of their jaw (Figure 4.6). If an incorrect size is used, it may result in trauma, laryngospasm and/or worsening of the airway obstruction.

The airway can be introduced directly, sliding it carefully over the tongue or alternatively, it can be introduced upside down initially and then rotated through 180 degrees, as for adults. In small children particularly, there is a risk of trauma to the delicate palatal structures and great care should be taken not to use any force. If this technique fails a laryngoscope blade or tongue depressor can be used to open the oropharynx and the airway can be introduced directly. Oropharyngeal airways are intended to be used only in unconscious patients. If the child is semi-conscious they may cough, vomit or develop laryngospasm. The latter insertion technique is particularly likely to cause coughing

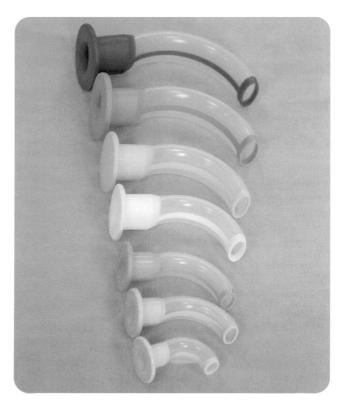

Figure 4.5 Oropharyngeal airways

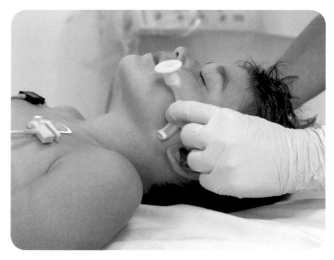

Figure 4.6 Sizing an oropharyngeal airway in a child

or gagging if the child is not deeply unconscious and the attempt should be abandoned if this occurs.

Following insertion of the oropharyngeal airway the child's airway patency should be reassessed by the 'look, listen and feel' approach and oxygen, if indicated, delivered appropriately.

Nasopharyngeal airways

The nasopharyngeal airway is a flexible tube that is designed to open a channel between the nostril and the nasopharynx. They are made of soft plastic or silicone, are bevelled at the insertion end and flanged at the outer end (Figure 4.7). The flange prevents the airway passing completely into the nasal passage. Tracheal tubes cut to the correct length may alternatively be used.

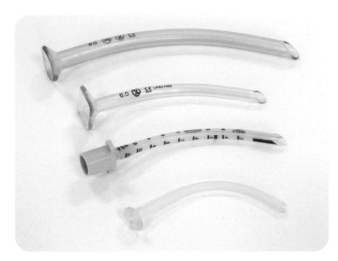

Figure 4.7 Nasopharyngeal airway

The correct length of nasopharyngeal airway should be estimated from the nostrils to the angle of the mandible. An appropriate tube size can be estimated by matching its diameter against the diameter of the child's anterior nares and when inserted it should not cause blanching of the nostril.

Once appropriately sized, the nasopharyngeal airway should be lubricated and introduced into the nostril. With a gentle rotating motion, the airway should be passed directly backwards and posteriorly along the floor of the nostril. The tube should not be directed upwards as this will cause trauma and bleeding (Figure 4.8). Following insertion of the nasopharyngeal airway, the child's airway patency should be reassessed by the 'look, listen and feel' approach and oxygen given if indicated.

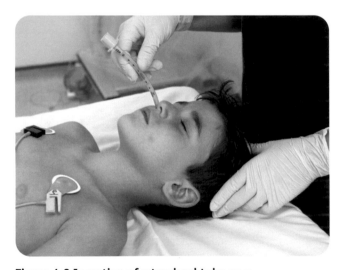

Figure 4.8 Insertion of a tracheal tube as a nasopharyngeal airway

Nasopharyngeal airways may be better tolerated by conscious children than oropharyngeal airways and are useful as adjuncts in the management of children who may improve their level of consciousness (e.g. the fitting child who is becoming less obtunded).

Their use is contraindicated in patients where basal skull fracture is suspected or if there is a coagulopathy.

Oxygen delivery and ventilatory support

Oxygen should be given as soon as it is available. Initially, this should be at the highest available concentration for all seriously ill children; concerns about oxygen toxicity should never prevent its use during initial resuscitation. The oxygen should be delivered through a flowmeter capable of delivering at least 15 L min⁻¹ (although this may be much higher when high flow nasal cannulae are used via a special flowmeter). It should ideally be warmed and humidified to minimise the risks of airway irritation and hypothermia. The method used to deliver the oxygen should be selected according to the child's clinical condition. Oxygen saturation levels should be monitored by pulse oximetry (SpO_2). When the child's condition has stabilised, the inspired oxygen concentration should be reduced, whilst monitoring SpO_2 to maintain adequate oxygenation. Table 4.1 shows the amounts of oxygen that is delivered for each oxygen delivery device.

Table 4.1 Oxygen delivery devices, flow rates and maximum inspired oxygen levels		
Device	**Flow rate**	**Maximum inspired**
Nasal prongs	Maximum 4 L min⁻¹	40%
Oxygen mask without reservoir	10–15 L min⁻¹	60%
Oxygen mask with reservoir	Must be enough to avoid reservoir collapse during inspiration (e.g. 12–15 L min⁻¹)	90%
Bag Mask Reservoir (BMV)	15 L min⁻¹	90%
High flow nasal cannulae	2–30 L min⁻¹*	100%

*Will vary between manufacturers

Oxygen administration methods

Oxygen mask with reservoir bag

This method is generally the preferred option in managing the seriously ill child who is breathing spontaneously. The flow of oxygen must be sufficiently high to ensure the reservoir bag does not collapse on inspiration (Figure 4.9). It is possible to deliver an oxygen concentration up to 90% with an oxygen delivery flow of 12–15 L min⁻¹.

These devices have three 'one-way' valves; one between the reservoir bag and the mask, and one on each side of the facemask over the inspiratory holes. They are designed so that when the child inhales, the valve between the mask and reservoir bag opens allowing oxygen to flow in to the mask, whilst the ones on either side of the mask close to prevent in-drawing of room air. When the child exhales, the valve between the mask and reservoir bag closes whilst the ones on either side of the mask open to allow escape of the child's expired breath (i.e. there is no rebreathing of gas).

When the side valves (or flaps) over the inspiratory holes are removed, a lower FiO_2 will be achieved, as room air will be drawn in to the mask as the child inhales.

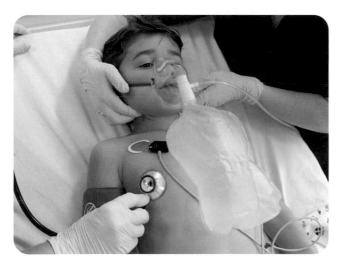

Figure 4.9 Non re-breathing oxygen mask with reservoir

Simple oxygen mask

A simple oxygen mask without a reservoir bag can deliver oxygen concentrations of up to 60% at flow rates of 10–15 L min^{-1}. Room air is entrained around the edges of the mask and through the holes in the mask so diluting the oxygen delivery.

'Blow-by' facial oxygen

Either the end of the oxygen tubing or a facemask can be held by the child's carer at a short distance from the child's face. This is a less-threatening method that can help to alleviate the child's fear and maximise their cooperation. However, the inspired concentration that can be delivered is low and inconsistent, so it is only suitable for children with mild respiratory compromise who cannot tolerate other methods of oxygen delivery. Oxygen flow rates need to be adjusted depending what the child will accept.

Nasal cannulae

This method can be useful in stable children of all ages, particularly in pre-school children. The delivery of oxygen via cannulae (or 'prongs') is dependent on oxygen flow and nasal resistance but the FiO_2 will be low and variable, so it is not suitable during resuscitation or when a high oxygen concentration is required. They are also not suitable for use in children with copious or tenacious nasal secretions, as they will easily become blocked. Flow rates should be kept below 4 L min^{-1} as higher flows are extremely irritating to the nasal passages and do not significantly increase oxygen delivery.

High flow nasal cannula oxygen

High flow nasal cannula oxygen (e.g. optiflow) is increasingly being used for critically ill patients, as it has the advantage of humidifying and warming the gases. It is also able to deliver a higher FiO_2 than standard nasal cannulae.

At high oxygen flow rates they are probably also able to deliver some positive end expiratory pressure (PEEP), which can be advantageous for hypoxic children (e.g. pneumonia, pulmonary contusion, and bronchiolitis).

Ventilation equipment

When providing positive pressure ventilation for an infant/child, the rescuer should aim for a respiratory rate of 12–20 breaths min^{-1}. In a newborn the rate should be 30 breaths min^{-1}. The volume delivered should be sufficient to produce visible chest expansion and breath sounds on auscultation. Continuous monitoring of the heart rate and SpO_2 should be undertaken as soon as practicable.

Mouth-to-mask devices

The pocket mask is widely used in resuscitation of apnoeic adults and the standard size may be suitable for use in larger children and adolescents. There is a 'paediatric' pocket mask available but it should be noted that this one size does not fit all infants and children, and an appropriate size of paediatric facemask should be substituted as soon as one becomes available. An appropriately sized facemask usually comes in conjunction with a manual ventilation device (e.g. self-inflating bag), and at that point the rescuer can stop using their own expired air.

When it is deemed appropriate for use (e.g. in an adolescent) the pocket mask is a device designed to minimise infection risks when delivering expired air ventilation. The device is made of transparent plastic with a one-way valve that directs the patient's expired breath away from the rescuer. An oxygen delivery port (which also has a one-way valve) is incorporated into some pocket masks, and allows supplemental oxygen to be administered.

Technique for mouth-to-mask ventilation

- Having assembled the pocket mask, the rescuer positions themselves behind the supine child.

- The child's head should be placed in an appropriate position (e.g. 'sniffing' position) to achieve a patent airway.

- Apply the mask over the child's mouth and nose, pressing down with the thumbs of both hands to create a seal.

- Lift the child's jaw upwards (jaw thrust) into the mask with the other fingers, taking care not to compress the soft tissues under the mandible.

- Blow through the mask's one-way valve until chest expansion is observed (Figure 4.10).

- Stop inflation and observe the chest falling.

- Repeat as appropriate.

- If chest expansion is not seen, assess whether this may be due to inadequate airway patency or a poor seal between the child's face and the mask, and correct as necessary.

- If the mask has an appropriate port and there is oxygen available, supplemental oxygen should be administered.

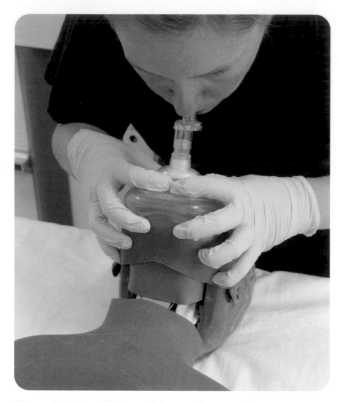

Figure 4.10 Ventilation with a pocket mask

Self-inflating bag-mask devices

In a child who has inadequate/absent breathing, maintenance of a patent airway is the first priority of management. Once this is achieved, adequate ventilation must be established. A self-inflating bag can be connected to a facemask, a tracheal tube or laryngeal mask airway when these are in place. The self-inflating bag can be used with or without a supplemental oxygen source, although in resuscitation situations, oxygen is almost always used in order to deliver ventilation with high inspired oxygen concentrations.

The self-inflating bag system consists of a bag which the operator squeezes to deliver a breath to the patient. Exhalation occurs through a one-way valve at the patient end of the bag, whilst the device automatically refills with air (and oxygen when attached) via an inlet(s) at the opposite end.

Used without supplemental oxygen a self-inflating bag system will ventilate with room air (21% oxygen). This can be increased to approximately 50% by attaching a high flow of oxygen to the gas inlet on the base of the bag. To increase this further, an oxygen reservoir bag is attached to the base. Together with a high flow of oxygen, this will enable the delivery of > 90% oxygen (Figure 4.11).

Self-inflating bags are available in three sizes (generally 250, 450–500 and 1600–2000 mL). The two smallest sizes usually have a pressure-limiting valve that prevents excessive inflation pressures that may cause barotrauma. The pressure limit is pre-determined by the manufacturers (usually 30–40 cm H_2O). During resuscitation higher than normal inflation pressures may be required and the pressure-limiting valve may need to be over-ridden. It is however, important to ensure that the child's airway is patent (e.g. check head positioning) before over-riding the valve. It should be noted that this device is also now being incorporated into some of the large bag sizes.

The smallest bag (250 mL) is intended for use in preterm neonates < 2.5 kg only. It is not appropriate for use in full term neonates and infants as it may be inadequate to support effective tidal volume.

The middle size of bag (450–500 mL) is generally the most appropriate for use in infants and pre-school aged children (Figures 4.11 and 4.12).

Self-inflating bags should not be used to deliver oxygen to spontaneously breathing patients; oxygen is only delivered when the one-way valve at the patient end of the bag is open and this only occurs when the bag is squeezed.

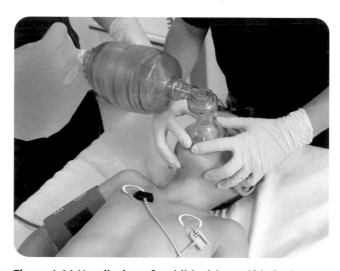

Figure 4.11 Ventilation of a child with a self-inflating bag-mask device

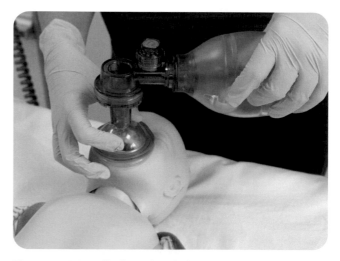

Figure 4.12 Ventilation of an infant with a self-inflating bag-mask device

The child's own respiratory efforts may not generate sufficient pressure to open the valve to receive oxygen. Children who are making adequate respiratory effort must therefore have oxygen administered by another method.

Facemask selection

These are the interface between the ventilation device and the child. They must be capable of providing a good seal over the mouth and nose whilst ensuring no pressure is applied over the eyes.

Masks are available in a variety of sizes and two basic types; anatomically shaped ones for older children and adults, and circular ones for infants and small children. The preferred mask is transparent (to allow rapid detection of secretions/vomitus and observation of the child's central colour) and should have a low dead space.

Correctly performed bag-mask ventilation (BMV) is an essential skill for all healthcare professionals who work with children. Whilst the operating principle of self-inflating bags is simple, they require skill to use them safely and effectively.

Hypoventilation can occur with poor technique (e.g. inadequate mask seal or incorrect head positioning) and is likely to have a negative effect on outcome.

Excessive ventilation volume can distend the stomach which reduces ventilation and increases the risk of gastro-oesophageal reflux and aspiration.

When self-inflating bags are used with a facemask, it can be difficult for a single rescuer to achieve an airtight seal whilst simultaneously using one hand to maintain a patent airway with a jaw thrust manoeuvre, and squeezing the bag with the other. A two-person technique (one person to maintain the airway and hold the mask in position, and the second to squeeze the bag) will usually overcome these difficulties.

Technique for bag-mask ventilation

- Having selected the appropriate size of bag and mask, the rescuer should stand behind the supine child.

- The oxygen supply should be connected at a high flow and the reservoir bag should be seen to inflate.

- If there is a second person available they should stand at one side of the child.

- The child's head should be placed in an appropriate position (e.g. 'neutral' position for an infant) to achieve a patent airway. A roll placed under the child's shoulders is often useful to assist in maintaining an appropriate airway position (unless contraindicated in trauma cases).

- Apply the mask over the child's mouth and nose, pressing down with the thumb and index finger of one hand (or both hands if two rescuers).

- Lift the child's jaw upwards (jaw thrust) into the mask with the other fingers, taking care not to compress the soft tissues underneath the mandible.

- Gently squeeze the bag until chest expansion is observed.

- Stop inflation and observe the chest falling.

- Repeat as appropriate.

- If chest expansion is not seen, assess whether this may be due to inadequate airway patency or a poor seal between the child's face and the mask, and correct as necessary.

Bag-mask ventilation frequently results in significant gastric distension, and therefore placement of a gastric tube should be undertaken as early as practicable.

T-piece and open-ended bag devices

This equipment is often employed by anaesthesia and critical care staff. It requires a continuous gas source for inflation of the bag, and therefore there must always be an appropriate self-inflating system immediately available in case there is a failure of the gas supply. This circuit does not have any valves and the bag has an open end. To achieve ventilation the end of the bag needs to be occluded and the bag squeezed. To prevent rebreathing a high gas flow is required (at least three times the minute ventilation of the patient, i.e. > 30 mL kg^{-1} x respiratory rate). This circuit can deliver 100% oxygen and can be used in spontaneously breathing children. The bag of this device gives some 'feeling' of the compliance of the lungs and allows some positive end expiratory pressure (PEEP) to be applied manually. The safe and effective use of this equipment requires considerable expertise and it should be utilised by experienced practitioners only.

Tracheal intubation

The indications for, and the techniques associated with, tracheal intubation are beyond the scope of the PILS course. The most important ventilation skill required of healthcare professionals dealing with children is effective BMV with a self-inflating bag device. The vast majority of children can be safely managed with BMV until expert help is available.

Summary learning

- Airway obstruction is commonly encountered in paediatric resuscitation (primary or secondary problem).

- Appropriate head positioning and simple airway adjuncts may be required to optimise airway patency.

- High concentration oxygen delivered in an appropriate manner is mandatory for seriously ill children.

- Correctly performed bag-mask ventilation (BMV) is an essential skill for all healthcare professionals who work with children.

My key take-home messages from this chapter

Management of circulation and drugs

Contents

- **Intravenous access in children during resuscitation**
- **Intraosseous access, advantages and disadvantages**
- **Fluid administration in resuscitation**
- **First-line resuscitation drugs**

Learning outcomes

To enable you to:

- **Understand the requirement for circulatory access**
- **Describe the advantages and potential complications of intraosseous access**
- **Understand the type and volume of fluids to be administered in the emergency situation**
- **Know the indications, dosages and actions of the first-line medications used in cardiorespiratory arrest**

Circulatory access

Once the airway is patent and adequate ventilation of the child is established, attention must be focused on circulation.

Establish circulatory access within the first few minutes of resuscitation in order that:

- medications (e.g. adrenaline) can be given

- fluids can be started

- blood samples can be obtained.

Circulatory access may be achieved via the intravenous (IV) or intraosseous (IO) routes. In cardiorespiratory arrest and/or severe shock states when peripheral circulation is severely compromised the IO route is the preferred method of gaining vascular access. The tracheal route is no longer recommended because of the variability in alveolar drug absorption.

For children who are unwell but remain responsive to pain, IV access is preferred over IO if possible, as infusions of fluids and drugs via the IO route can be painful. If there is an IV cannula already in situ, check its patency before use otherwise insert the largest possible IV cannula in peripheral veins (e.g. the antecubital fossa, the long saphenous vein or the back of the hand (or feet in smaller children)).

The use of scalp veins during resuscitation is not advisable owing to the risk of extravasation leading to potential tissue necrosis. Their use may also interfere with the management of the airway and ventilation. If the child requires chest compressions these should not be interrupted by access attempts or other procedures apart from defibrillation.

Intraosseous access

In cardiorespiratory arrest, the IO route is the emergency circulatory access route of choice. Placement of an IO cannula involves insertion of a needle through the skin, periosteum and cortex of a bone, into the medullary cavity. The IO route should be **the first choice** in any situation where the child's clinical status is severely compromised (i.e. they are in a decompensated state) or they have suffered a cardiorespiratory arrest. The main advantages of IO access are:

- The relative ease and speed of insertion.

- It can be used to deliver all resuscitation fluids, medications and blood-derived products.

- It allows rapid adequate plasma concentration of medications similar to that of central venous administration (more rapid and reliable than that achieved through a peripheral IV).

- It permits bone marrow aspiration, which can be used for analysis. In this situation, the laboratory should be informed as the fat in a marrow sample may cause damage to auto-analysers.

Insertion of an intraosseous cannula

Before undertaking this procedure, the appropriate equipment must be available and there should be no contraindications to IO insertion.

Insertion site – anatomical landmarks

The usual site for insertion of an IO cannula is 2–3 cm below the tuberosity on the anteromedial surface of the tibia (Figure 5.1). Other sites that can be used include the lower end of the tibia (approximately 1–3 cm above the medial malleolus) or on the centro-medial aspect of the distal femur (1–2 cm above patella and 1–2 cm medial to midline). These sites specifically avoid the growth plates of the bones.

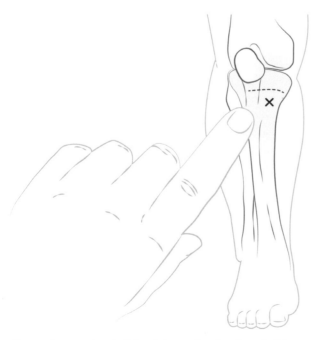

Figure 5.1 Proximal tibia IO insertion landmark (X)

Contraindications

Contraindications to the insertion of an IO needle include osteogenesis imperfecta ('brittle bone' disease) and haemophilia or other known coagulopathies.
IO cannulation should not be through an area of infected skin or wounds. Fractured bones must not be used, nor should the cannula be inserted into a bone immediately distal to a fracture site, as this may predispose to the development of compartment syndrome.

Equipment required

1. IO cannulae

There are several designs of manually inserted IO cannulae available commercially. They come in a variety of sizes. Generally, it is recommended that size 18 gauge is used for a newborn–6 months of age, 16 gauge for a child between 6–18 months, and 14 gauge for children > 18 months.

Powered IO needle devices are becoming more popular and the EZ-IO device has become the device of choice for many hospitals as it requires minimal practice and training and results show it to be a safe and rapid means of obtaining IO access. Most resuscitation trolleys should carry a manual needle as well as a powered device in case of equipment failure.

2. Alcohol-based skin preparation solution to minimise the risk of infection.

3. Three-way tap with integrated IV extension tubing primed with 0.9% saline and attached to a syringe to allow for flushing of medications.

4. Syringe.

5. Emergency medications and/or fluids.

6. Local anaesthetic agent. If the child is still conscious, this should be considered to minimise pain, along the intended track of the IO cannula.

Potential complications

Although these are uncommon, complications can occur. These include:

- Extravasation: true extravasation ('tissuing') of an IO cannula is uncommon. However, transient swelling of subcutaneous tissue is commonly seen as fluid leaks from the marrow cavity into surrounding tissues. If the swelling does not rapidly subside or there is concern that the cannula is misplaced, the rescuer should withdraw a small amount of fluid; this aspirate should be blood stained if the cannula is in the correct place.

- Embolism: There is a small risk (estimated at < 1%) of fat or bone marrow embolism

- Infection: (e.g. osteomyelitis or cellulitis)

- Compartment syndrome

- Skin necrosis

- Fracture

The potential for any of the listed complications other than fracture can be minimised by removing the cannula as soon as alternative secure intravenous access has been obtained.

Fluid administration for volume resuscitation

Intravascular fluids are primarily administered to restore circulatory volume and ensure adequate perfusion of vital organs.

During cardiorespiratory arrest, hypovolaemia is often a primary contributory factor and fluid resuscitation may play a critical part in achieving return of spontaneous circulation.

The administration of fluids is also indicated for any child exhibiting signs of circulatory failure (e.g. decreased skin perfusion, prolonged capillary refill time, hypotension). The only children in whom caution is advised are those in suspected cardiogenic shock where the heart is unable to deal with the volume load or those with diabetic ketoacidosis.

Fluid volumes

During the resuscitation of a child with compromised circulation due to hypovolaemia (including sepsis and anaphylaxis), initial resuscitation fluid is administered as a bolus of 20 mL kg^{-1}. The child's circulatory status should then be reassessed and if signs of circulatory failure persist, this should be repeated. Signs of over-transfusion are moist sounds ('crackles') at the lung bases and jugular venous distension in children or liver distension in infants.

If circulatory failure is due to other causes, such as cardiac failure, a smaller initial volume (10 mL kg^{-1}) should be used. The effect of each smaller bolus should be carefully assessed to ensure that fluid administration is not causing worsening of the circulation (e.g. crackles at the lung bases and size of liver edge). The fluid bolus size in trauma is also 10 mL kg^{-1} followed by careful clinical reassessment because excessive fluid administration in trauma is associated with increased morbidity.

Fluids are indicated during cardiorespiratory arrest if hypovolaemic shock is a likely cause of the arrest. However, excessive amounts should be avoided as fluid overload is counterproductive and may be harmful in post resuscitation states.

The aim in the management of hypovolaemic shock is to prevent the onset of decompensated circulatory failure, as this may lead to irreversible cardiorespiratory failure and death. Measurement of blood pressure is of little help in determining circulatory status as it remains normal in compensated circulatory failure and only starts to drop as decompensation develops.

The principles of management adhere to ABCDE (airway, breathing, circulation, disability, exposure) with fluid administration forming part of the 'C' phase of resuscitation.

Types of fluid

In the initial phase of resuscitation, isotonic salt solutions should be used. There are no clear advantages between using crystalloid or colloid solutions. Glucose containing solutions (such as dextrose saline) should never be used for volume replacement as they can cause hyponatraemia and hyperglycaemia, which in turn, can lead to further fluid loss.

Crystalloids

Examples of appropriate resuscitation crystalloids include:

- 0.9% saline

- Ringer's lactate

- Hartmann's solution

Crystalloids are cheap, readily available and do not cause allergic reactions. They are however, less efficient than colloids at increasing circulating volume within the intravascular space, as they rapidly move into the surrounding interstitium; only 50–75% of the administered volume remains in the intravascular compartment. Therefore, to correct the initial circulatory deficit volume, 1.5–2 times this volume has to be infused; this may be poorly tolerated in children with underlying cardiac or respiratory disease, and pulmonary oedema may occur.

Infusion of fluids containing potassium must be avoided, particularly in children with anuria or oliguria, as hyperkalaemia could arise.

Glucose solutions should never be used for volume expansion as they can cause hyperglycaemia, resulting in osmotic diuresis. This increases urine production and so increases circulatory volume loss. Glucose solutions should only be used to correct hypoglycaemia following measurement of blood sugar levels: 2 mL kg^{-1} of 10% glucose is given and the patient's blood sugar should be re-measured shortly afterwards to ensure it is within the normal range. In the newborn 2.5 mL kg^{-1} of 10% glucose may be given initially to correct hypoglycaemia.

Colloids

Examples of colloids include:

- Human albumin (4.5%) solution

- Fresh frozen plasma (FFP)

- Gelatin solutions (e.g. Gelofusin)

Colloids are relatively expensive and less readily available than crystalloids. Colloids should be not be used in anaphylaxis because of the potential risk of allergic reaction. The main reason for considering the use of colloids in resuscitation is that they remain in the vascular space for longer, and may therefore increase the circulatory volume more efficiently than crystalloids.

Blood products

The administration of blood products is reserved for situations where there is a specific indication for their use (i.e. blood loss or coagulopathy).

If the infusion of 20 mL kg^{-1} (i.e 10 mL kg^{-1} bolus x 2) does not improve the circulatory status of a child who has suffered trauma, transfusion of blood must be considered, as well as urgent surgical referral.

In an emergency, Group O Rhesus-negative 'flying squad' blood or type specific uncross-matched blood may be used for transfusion until fully cross-matched blood is available.

Fresh frozen plasma should only be used in resuscitation situations for the treatment of specific coagulation abnormalities.

The risks of blood product administration must always be borne in mind.

First-line resuscitation medications

Only a few medications are indicated during the initial resuscitation phase of a child in cardiorespiratory arrest. Administration of medications should be considered only after adequate ventilation and chest compressions have been established, and in the case of a shockable arrhythmia (VF or pVT), following delivery of the first three defibrillation shocks.

For safety reasons, as well as speed and ease of use, the use of pre-filled medication syringes is advocated.

All medications administered should be followed by a flush of 2–5 mL 0.9% saline to ensure they reach the circulation and to minimise the risks of interactions with any other medications or fluids administered via the same cannula. All medications and fluids should be recorded as they are administered and then documented at the end of the resuscitation attempt.

Adrenaline

Indication for use:

- cardiorespiratory arrest of any aetiology

- bradycardia < 60 min^{-1} with decompensated circulatory shock after the initial steps to restore satisfactory oxygenation and ventilation have been taken

- first line inotrope in fluid resistant shock

- hypotension with anaphylaxis

It should be given as soon as circulatory access has been achieved in non-shockable rhythms and after **the 3rd shock in shockable rhythms.**

Dosage: in cardiorespiratory arrest or bradycardia with decompensated circulatory failure 10 mcg kg^{-1} (or 0.1 mL kg^{-1} of 1:10 000 solution). This is repeated every 3–5 min as necessary.

Actions: adrenaline is an endogenous, directly acting sympathomimetic amine with both alpha and beta adrenergic activity. In the dose used in resuscitation, adrenaline produces vasoconstriction, which results in increased cerebral and coronary perfusion pressure. It also increases myocardial contractility and may facilitate defibrillation success.

Adrenaline frequently causes tachycardia and may produce or exacerbate ventricular ectopics.

Higher doses of adrenaline (100 mcg kg^{-1}) administered by the vascular route are not recommended routinely as they do not improve survival or neurological outcome after cardiorespiratory arrest.

Amiodarone

Indication for use: refractory ventricular fibrillation (VF) or pulseless ventricular tachycardia (pVT). If VF or pVT persists after the 3rd defibrillation shock, a dose of amiodarone should be given with adrenaline. This can be repeated after the 5th shock if defibrillation is still unsuccessful.

Dosage: 5 mg kg^{-1}.

Actions: amiodarone is a membrane-stabilising anti-arrhythmic medication that increases the duration of the action potential and refractory period in both atrial and ventricular myocardium. Atrioventricular conduction is also slowed, and a similar effect is seen in accessory pathways. Amiodarone has a mild negative inotropic action and causes peripheral vasodilatation through non-competitive alpha-blocking effects. The hypotension that occurs with IV amiodarone is related to the rate of delivery and is due more to the solvent (Polysorbate 80 and benzyl alcohol), which causes histamine release, rather than the drug itself. The oral form is not well absorbed but the intravenous form has been successfully used for tachyarrhythmia management.

Precaution: amiodarone should be given as a pre-filled syringe preparation or diluted in 5% glucose. Ideally, it should be administered via a central vascular (IV or IO) route as it can cause thrombophlebitis. If it has to be given peripherally it should be liberally flushed with 0.9% saline or 5% glucose.

Sodium bicarbonate

This is not a first-line resuscitation medication. Studies have shown that the routine use of sodium bicarbonate does not improve outcome.

Indication for use: The routine use of sodium bicarbonate is not recommended. It may be considered in prolonged arrest and it has a specific role in management of hyperkalaemia and the arrhythmias associated with tricyclic antidepressant or some inborn errors of metabolism.

Dosage: the initial dose is 1 mmol kg^{-1}. This equates to 1 mL kg^{-1} of 8.4% solution, although in newborns and infants < 3 months the weaker concentration (i.e. 4.2%) solution should be used to limit the osmotic load.

The decision to give further doses should be based on blood gas analysis.

Actions: sodium bicarbonate is administered to reverse metabolic acidosis. However, as it elevates $PaCO_2$ levels, the administration of sodium bicarbonate may worsen existing respiratory acidosis, a possible cause of the cardiorespiratory arrest. It may also cause paradoxical intracellular acidosis, thus worsening cellular function (e.g. myocardial dysfunction may be induced by the acidosis within myocardial cells). Some of the specific effects of sodium bicarbonate administration include:

- carbon dioxide production which diffuses into cells and exacerbates the intracellular acidosis

- left displacement of the oxyhaemoglobin dissociation curve inhibiting oxygen release to the tissues

- intracellular shift of potassium

- hypernatraemia due to the high, osmotically active, sodium content

- lowered VF threshold

- decreased plasma calcium.

The potential negative effects of sodium bicarbonate outweigh any benefits unless the metabolic acidosis is severe, and even then it should be used with caution.

Precautions: arterial blood gas analysis does not reflect venous or tissue pH and should be interpreted with caution. Care should also be taken to ensure that an adequate flush of 0.9% saline is given between delivery of sodium bicarbonate and any other medications via the same cannula, as incompatibilities may occur.

Atropine

Indication for use: Bradycardia resulting from vagal stimulation. There is no evidence that atropine has any benefit in asphyxial bradycardia or asystole and its routine use has been removed from the advanced life support algorithms.

Dosage: 20 mcg kg^{-1}.

This dose may be repeated but, once the vagus nerve has been fully blocked, there is no further beneficial effect.

Actions: Atropine blocks the effect of the vagus nerve on the sinoatrial (SA) and atrioventricular (AV) nodes, increasing sinus automaticity, facilitating AV node conduction and increasing heart rate. The functions of the vagus nerve include pupillary constriction, contraction of the gut and production of salivary and gastro-intestinal secretions. During resuscitation, atropine may be of benefit in treating bradycardia which accompanies actions that result in vagal stimulation such as laryngoscopy.

Summary learning

- **Intraosseous access is the circulatory route of choice in cardiorespiratory arrest and decompensated circulatory failure.**

- **Fluid resuscitation starts with 20 mL kg^{-1} boluses.**

- **After each fluid bolus, the child's condition must be reassessed.**

- **The role of medications is secondary to effective ventilation and chest compressions (and, if indicated, defibrillation) in cardiorespiratory arrest.**

- **The main medication used in cardiorespiratory arrest is IV or IO adrenaline, which can be repeated as necessary every 3–5 minutes.**

- **Amiodarone is used in refractory VF or pVT after the 3rd and 5th shock.**

My key take-home messages from this chapter

pILS

Rhythm recognition

Contents

- **The normal ECG**
- **Abnormal ECG traces and clinical correlation**
- **How to manage common tachy and bradyarrhythmias seen in acutely unwell children**

Learning outcomes

To enable you to:

- **Describe the normal electrocardiogram (ECG) trace**
- **Recognise cardiac rhythms associated with cardiorespiratory arrest**
- **Describe the management of bradycardia**
- **Differentiate between sinus tachycardia (ST) and supraventricular tachycardia (SVT)**
- **Management priorities in children with compensated and decompensated tachyarrhythmias**

ECG monitoring

Once optimal ventilation and oxygenation have been established, all seriously ill children should have their ECG monitored continuously via lead II and at least one 12 lead ECG should be performed. This facilitates the observation of heart rate changes, which are important indicators of the response to treatments, or the evolution of the disease process. It should be remembered that normal heart rates vary for physiological reasons (e.g. pain, pyrexia and wakefulness), and with age (Table 6.1).

Table 6.1: Heart rate ranges (beats min^{-1})			
Age	Mean	Awake	Deep sleep
Newborn – 3 months	140	85–205	80–140
3 months – 2 years	130	100–180	75–160
2 – 10 years	80	60–140	60–90
> 10 years	75	60–100	50–90

Acute illness in children can result in cardiac arrhythmias. Much less frequently, the cardiac arrhythmia may be the trigger for the episode of acute illness. In these cases there is commonly a underlying cardiac anatomical anomaly or a reason for electrolyte disturbance causing abnormal cardiac electrical conductivity.

Examples include:

- acquired cardiac disease (e.g. cardiomyopathy, myocarditis)

- congenital heart disease or following cardiac surgery

- electrolyte disturbances (e.g. renal disease).

Additionally, some medications (in therapeutic or toxic amounts) may also cause arrhythmias (e.g. digoxin, beta-blockers, tricyclic antidepressants).

By monitoring the ECG, it is possible to detect those arrhythmias that are (or have the potential to become) life-threatening.

Basic electrocardiography

The ECG trace represents electrical activity within the heart, and not the effectiveness of myocardial contraction or tissue perfusion. The child's clinical status needs to be considered alongside the ECG trace: **treat the patient not the monitor.**

When evaluating the ECG, possible artefacts may occur; detachment of ECG electrodes or leads can simulate asystole, whilst vibrations transmitted to the leads (e.g. during patient transportation) can mimic ventricular fibrillation (VF).

A normal ECG complex consists of a P wave, a QRS complex and a T wave (Figure 6.1).

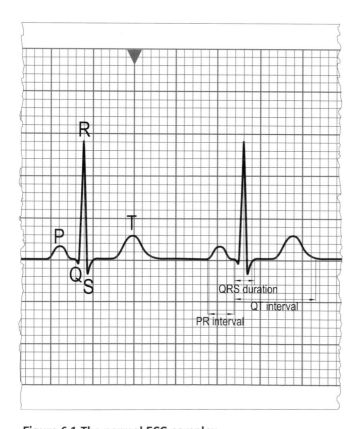

Figure 6.1 The normal ECG complex

The P wave represents electrical depolarisation of the atria. The time taken for depolarisation to pass through the atria, atrio-ventricular (AV) node and His-Purkinje system to the ventricles (Figure 6.2) is represented by the P-R interval. The QRS complex represents depolarisation of the ventricular myocardium. Ventricular repolarisation, in preparation for the next impulse, is represented by the ST segment and the T wave. A prolonged QT interval is a risk factor for arrhythmias and sudden death.

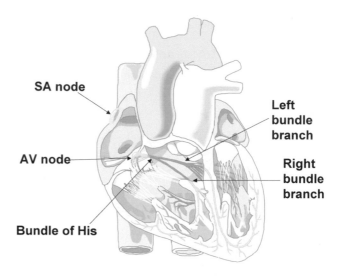

Figure 6.2 Electrical conduction through the heart

Cardiac rhythm disturbances

The approach to managing a child with a cardiac rhythm disturbance is summarised in Figure 6.3. This approach is based on determining the following 4 factors:

1. Presence or absence of circulation (i.e. a central pulse and other 'signs of life' (chapter 3)).

2. Clinical status – compensated (haemodynamically stable) or decompenstated (haemodynamically unstable).

3. Heart rate (bradycardia or tachycardia).

4. Width of QRS complexes on ECG (i.e. narrow or broad).

1. Presence of central pulse

Adopting the ABCDE approach, the rescuer must quickly establish the absence or presence of cardiac output (i.e. 'signs of life' and a palpable central pulse).

Absent pulse

The absence of 'signs of life' and no palpable central pulse indicates cardiorespiratory arrest. BLS should be started immediately. The rhythms associated with cardiorespiratory arrest are:

- asystole (or severe bradycardia)

- pulseless electrical activity (PEA)

- ventricular fibrillation (VF)

- pulseless ventricular tachycardia (pVT).

The commonest cardiorespiratory arrest arrhythmia in paediatrics is asystole (generally preceded by progressive bradycardia). The term PEA describes the situation where there is organised electrical activity displayed on the ECG monitor but no cardiac output. The principles of managing both asystole and PEA are the provision of effective CPR, administration of adrenaline and the treatment of any underlying problems.

Both VF and pVT are less common in children, but more likely in those with underlying cardiac disease. The priority of management in these arrhythmias is effective CPR and rapid defibrillation. VF and pVT may also occur as a secondary rhythm during reperfusion of the myocardium during a cardiorespiratory arrest.

The management of cardiorespiratory arrest is outlined in Chapter 8.

Pulse present

If there is a central pulse present, determine whether or not the child is compensated (haemodynamically stable) or decompensated (haemodynamically unstable).

2. Clinical status

Compensated circulatory failure

The child with compensated circulatory failure, who is haemodynamically stable, must be monitored, including an ECG. If the ECG displays an arrhythmia, the child may need treatment, but it is reasonable to await expert help such as from a paediatric cardiologist. Preparations should be made to intervene (along the principles described below) should the child deteriorate and become decompensated.

Decompensated circulatory failure

The child who is decompensated (haemodynamically unstable) should be monitored and, if the ECG displays a life-threatening arrhythmia, the immediate interventions that may be required are outlined below. Urgent expert help must also be sought. This should include an anaesthetist or a paediatric intensivist as sedation or anaesthesia is required to manage a conscious child requiring cardioversion.

3. Heart rate

Both bradycardia and tachycardia are relatively common in paediatrics. Their defining heart rates are listed in Table 6.2.

Table 6.2: Bradycardia and tachycardia heart rates (beats min⁻¹)		
Age	Bradycardia	Tachycardia
< 1 year	< 80*	> 180
> 1 year	< 60	> 160

*although 80 min⁻¹ is defining rate for bradycardia in an infant chest compressions are not indicated until the heart rate is < 60 min⁻¹.

Bradycardia

Bradycardia may be due to hypoxia, acidosis and respiratory or circulatory failure, and it may be a pre-terminal event prior to cardiorespiratory arrest.

A bradycardic child with signs of decompensation or a child with a rapidly dropping heart rate associated with poor systemic perfusion requires immediate oxygenation (airway opening, 100% oxygen administration and positive pressure ventilation as necessary). If the heart rate remains < 60 min⁻¹ (all ages) and the child has decompensated circulatory failure, chest compressions must also be started. The cause of the bradycardia must be sought and treatment directed at the underlying cause.

By far the commonest causes of bradycardia in infants and children are hypoxia and vagal stimulation. Less commonly, hypothermia and hypoglycaemia can slow conduction through cardiac tissues and result in bradycardia. Infants and children with a history of heart surgery are at increased risk of sick sinus syndrome or heart block secondary to injury of the AV node or other parts of the conduction system.

Atropine is indicated when increased vagal tone is the cause of the bradycardia (e.g. induced by tracheal intubation or suctioning); otherwise adrenaline is the medication of choice but only once oxygenation has been restored and the HR remains < 60 min⁻¹ with circulatory failure. Very occasionally, in a child with congenital heart disease, the bradycardia is due to complete heart block, and emergency cardiac pacing is required. Pacing is not indicated in children with bradycardia secondary to hypoxic/ischaemic myocardial insult or respiratory failure.

Tachycardia

An elevated heart rate is frequently the normal physiological response to anxiety, pain or pyrexia. This is **sinus tachycardia (ST)** and is managed by treating the primary cause.

Other causes of ST include:

- respiratory conditions; early hypoxia, hypercapnia, obstructed airway and pneumothorax

- circulatory conditions; hypovolaemia, cardiac failure, anaphylaxis or sepsis, pulmonary hypertension

- miscellaneous causes; drugs, seizures.

The other cause of tachycardia is **a tachyarrhythmia**, either supraventricular tachycardia (SVT) or ventricular tachycardia (VT). Of these, SVT is far more common in children. The priority of management is to establish whether or not the child is stable, or if they are displaying signs of circulatory decompensation. If the child is in a compensated state, expert help should be sought for definitive management.

The child who has decompensated circulatory failure requires chemical or electrical cardioversion whilst ABCDE is continually assessed and appropriately supported.

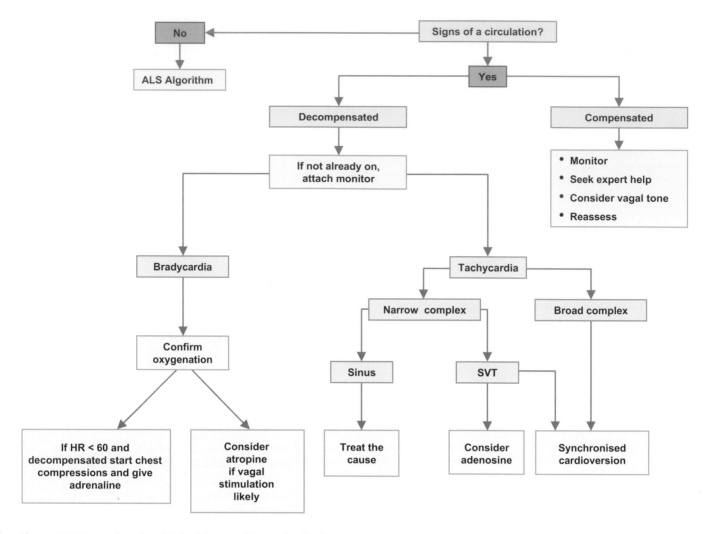

Figure 6.3 Managing the child with a cardiac arrhythmia

4. Width of QRS complexes

In children with a tachycardia the most important thing to establish is whether this is **ST** or an abnormal rhythm **(tachyarrhythmia).** The history and clinical examination are key in determining this. The ECG features and width of the QRS complexes can also be helpful but it is always the child's clinical status that determines the urgency of management, regardless of the type of arrhythmia.

Narrow QRS complex tachycardia

Both ST (Figure 6.4) and SVT (Figure 6.5) have narrow QRS complexes, making it potentially difficult to differentiate between them. The clinical and ECG differences that help to make this distinction are listed in Table 6.3.

Broad QRS complex tachycardia

In children, broad complex tachycardia is uncommon; if present, the cause is usually SVT with abnormal conduction making the complex broad. However, if uncertain, the rhythm should be treated as though it is VT as this has more immediately serious consequences if inadequately treated (i.e. it can deteriorate to VF or pVT).

VT is usually found in a child who has underlying cardiac disease.

VT is broad complex, regular rhythm. The p waves are either absent or unrelated to the QRS complexes (Figure 6.6). It can present with or without a pulse; pVT is managed in the same manner as VF (i.e. it presents with cardiorespiratory arrest and needs CPR and urgent defibrillation).

The management of VT with a pulse involves urgent expert help, as it has the potential to rapidly deteriorate to pVT or VF. The ongoing management of these children may involve electrical synchronised cardioversion or chemical cardioversion (i.e. with Amiodarone). **An anaesthetist should be present** (in addition to a cardiologist if available) because amiodarone can cause profound hypotension and may result in the rapid onset of decompensated circulatory failure and if electrical cardioversion is required anaesthesia may be necessary.

Supraventricular tachycardia

SVT is the most common primary cardiac arrhythmia observed in children. It is a paroxysmal, regular rhythm usually with narrow QRS complexes, caused by a re-entry

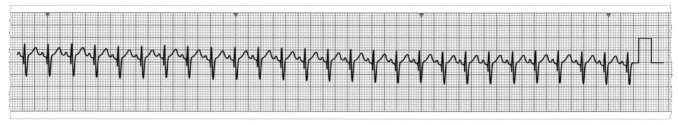

Figure 6.4 Sinus tachycardia rhythm strip

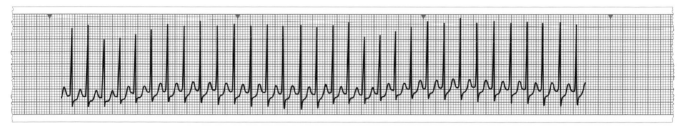

Figure 6.5 Supraventricular tachycardia rhythm strip

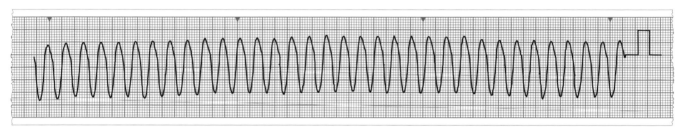

Figure 6.6 Ventricular tachycardia rhythm strip

mechanism through an accessory pathway or the atrioventricular conduction system. A heart rate of > 220 min^{-1} in infants or > 180 min^{-1} in children older than 1 year is highly suggestive of SVT. The other features that help to differentiate SVT from ST are listed in Table 6.3.

Management of SVT

Once a diagnosis of SVT is made, the child's clinical status will determine the management. As described previously, a child with **compensated** circulatory status should be referred for expert help. They may suggest that vagal manoeuvres be performed, as stimulation of the vagus nerve may slow atrioventricular conduction and result in a return to normal sinus rhythm.

Vagal manoeuvres

In infants and small children, vagal manoeuvres can be performed by soaking a flannel in ice cold water, and then placing it briefly over their face. In cooperative children, a Valsalva manoeuvre can be induced by asking the child to blow through a drinking straw. A variation on this is to blow through the outlet of a syringe in an effort to expel the plunger.

Adenosine

If intravascular access is already established in a conscious, compensated child with SVT, chemical cardioversion with adenosine may be possible. Adenosine should be given rapidly via a vein as close to the heart as possible, as it is metabolised by red blood cells as soon as it enters the bloodstream. A rapid bolus of 0.1 mg kg^{-1}

Table 6.3 Clinical and ECG differences between ST and SVT		
	ST	**SVT**
History	Clues (e.g. pyrexia, fluid or blood loss)	Non specific Previous arrhythmia
Heart rate (beats min^{-1})	Infant < 220 min^{-1} Child < 180 min^{-1}	Infant > 220 min^{-1} Child > 180 min^{-1}
P wave	Present and normal (N.B. not clearly seen at heart rates > 200 min^{-1})	Absent or abnormal
Beat-to-beat variability (R – R)	Yes – can be altered with stimulation	None
Onset and end	Gradual	Abrupt

should be followed with a flush of 2–5 mL 0.9% saline. If this dose is ineffective, it can be doubled (i.e. 0.2 mg kg^{-1}). The maximum dosages are 6 mg for the first attempt and 12 mg for the second. **Caution:** Adenosine can precipitate severe bronchospasm. It causes unpleasant feelings of impending doom in the child and should ideally only be given under the guidance of a paediatric cardiologist or intensivist.

Adenosine should be used with caution in heart transplant recipients and asthmatics.

Cardioversion

The procedure for undertaking synchronised electrical cardioversion is described in Chapter 7. It is the procedure of choice for decompensated children with SVT, particularly if they are unconscious. A general anaesthetic or deep sedation will be required if the child is conscious. The first shock should be delivered at the energy level of 1 J kg^{-1}, and the second (if required) at 2 J kg^{-1}. If the SVT fails to convert after a second shock, amiodarone maybe recommended before further shocks are delivered. This should ideally be under the guidance of a paediatric cardiologist or paediatric intensivist.

Summary learning

- **Life-threatening cardiac arrhythmias are more frequently the result, rather than the cause, of acute illness.**

- **The child's clinical status dictates management priorities – treat the patient not the monitor.**

- **The cause of the arrhythmia should be sought and treated.**

My key take-home messages from this chapter

Defibrillation and cardioversion

Contents

- **Definition of defibrillation**
- **Types of defibrillators**
- **Sequence of actions for defibrillation and cardioversion**
- **Defibrillation safety**

Learning outcomes

To enable you to:

- **Describe the indications for defibrillation and cardioversion**
- **Understand how to safely deliver an electrical shock using either a manual or automated external defibrillator (AED)**
- **Discuss the factors influencing the likelihood of successful defibrillation/cardioversion**

Incidence of shockable arrhythmias

Although the initial rhythm in a paediatric cardiorespiratory arrest is far more likely to be asystole or pulseless electrical activity (PEA) than ventricular fibrillation (VF) or pulseless ventricular tachycardia (pVT), a shockable rhythm is present in up to 27% of paediatric in-hospital arrests at some point during the resuscitation. When a shockable rhythm is present, the likelihood of a successful outcome is critically dependent on rapid, safe defibrillation.

A defibrillator can also be used in the management of a child with circulatory compromise due to VT with a pulse or supraventricular tachycardia (SVT) (Chapter 6). In these situations, the machine is used to perform synchronised DC (direct current) cardioversion, which is also described in this chapter.

Defibrillation

Defibrillation is the generic term used to describe the procedure of passing an electrical current across the myocardium with the intention of inducing global myocardial depolarisation and restoring organised spontaneous electrical activity. This electrical current may be delivered asynchronously when there is no cardiac output (in VF or pVT), or it may be synchronised with the R wave when there is an output (in SVT or VT with a pulse), the latter being called cardioversion.

The energy dosage should cause minimal myocardial injury. The electrical current delivered to the heart depends on the selected energy (in joules) and the resistance to current flow (thoracic impedance). If the impedance is high, the energy requirement will be increased.

Factors determining thoracic impedance

The factors that potentially affect thoracic impedance and therefore the energy required include:

- defibrillator pads/paddles size

- interface between pads/paddles and the child's skin

- positioning of the pads/paddles on the chest wall

- chest wall thickness and obesity.

Types of defibrillators

Defibrillators are either automatic (i.e. automated external defibrillators (AEDs)) or manually operated. They may be capable of delivering either monophasic or biphasic shocks. AEDs are pre-set for all parameters including the energy dose.

Manual defibrillators capable of delivering the full range of energy requirements for newborns through to adults must be available within all healthcare facilities caring for children at risk of cardiorespiratory arrest.

In children requiring cardioversion (e.g. a child with circulatory failure from SVT) a manual defibrillator should be used.

Monophasic defibrillators

Monophasic defibrillators are no longer manufactured but may remain in use. They deliver a unipolar (one way) current.

Biphasic defibrillators

There are various types of biphasic waveform but there is no data to support one being superior to another. There is however, good evidence that biphasic defibrillators are more effective than monophasic ones. A biphasic defibrillator delivers a current that flows in a positive direction, and then in reverse for a specified duration. First shock efficacy for long-lasting VF/pVT is better with biphasic than monophasic waveforms. Biphasic waves also appear to cause less post-shock cardiac dysfunction.

Paddles or pads?

Manual defibrillation is now more commonly performed using self-adhesive pads (i.e. 'hands free' defibrillation) rather than using manual defibrillator paddles. Self-adhesive pads are safe, effective and generally preferable to defibrillator paddles. A major advantage of using self-adhesive pads is that they allow the rescuer to defibrillate from a safe distance, rather than having to lean across the patient; this is particularly important when access to the patient is restricted in a confined space. They deliver the shock more rapidly and with less interruption to CPR as the machine can be charged whilst chest compressions are in progress.

Position of self-adhesive pads

Self-adhesive pads should be placed on the child's chest in a position that 'brackets' the heart to facilitate the flow of electrical current across it. The standard positioning is to place one pad just below the right clavicle to the right of the sternum and the other in the mid-axillary line on the left of the chest (Figure 7.1). Alternative pad position is anterior-posterior (Figure 7.2). Using this position, some defibrillators will provide feedback on the quality of chest compressions (rate, recoil and depth).

When using self-adhesive pads, it is essential to ensure that they do not touch each other. Selection of appropriate pads relating to the child's size/age may also be necessary, although this varies between manufacturers. The pads should be smoothed onto the child's chest ensuring that no air is trapped underneath as this will increase impedance and reduce the efficiency of the defibrillation shock. Although the pads are generally labelled right and left or have a diagram of their correct positioning on the chest, it does not matter if they have been reversed. Therefore if they have accidentally been placed the wrong way round they should be left in place and not repositioned. Repositioning results in time wasting and the self-adhesive pads may stick less effectively.

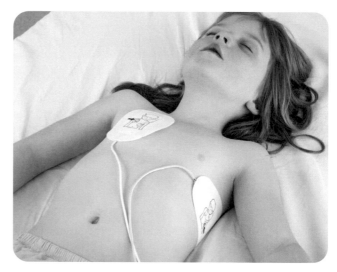

Figure 7.1 Self-adhesive defibrillation pads in position on a child

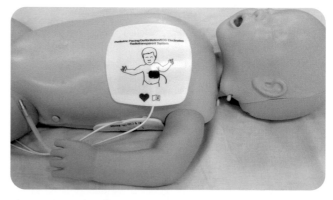

Figure 7.2 Self adhesive pads in the anterior-posterior position on an infant

Energy levels

Manual defibrillators

Manual defibrillators (Figure 7.3) have several advantages over AEDs and therefore must be readily available in all healthcare settings where children at risk of cardiorespiratory arrest may be cared for, even when AEDs are located nearby. The advantages include:

- ability to alter energy levels

- trained operators can diagnose arrhythmias and, when appropriate, deliver shocks more rapidly (with AEDs this diagnosis must await the results of the machine's rhythm analysis)

- additional facilities permit other treatments (e.g. synchronised cardioversion or external pacing).

When using a manual defibrillator an energy dose of 4 J per kg body weight (4 J kg^{-1}) should be used for all shocks, regardless of whether they are monophasic or biphasic waveforms. In a large child, the adult dosages should not be exceeded.

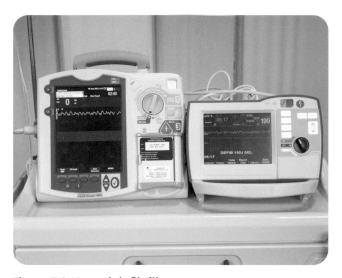

Figure 7.3 Manual defibrillators

Automated external defibrillators

These machines are now widely available including through Public Access Defibrillation (PAD) schemes as fully or semi-automated devices (Figure 7.4). They are safe, reliable and sophisticated and are increasingly used by health professionals and lay rescuers.

If there is any likelihood of use in infants and small children check with the manufacturer that the machine is suitable. Machines with paediatric attenuation devices are preferable.

The AED will analyse the patient's ECG rhythm, determine whether a defibrillation shock is indicated and facilitate the delivery of a shock. In the semi-automated models, follow the AED prompts and press the relevant button.

Some of the models available to healthcare professionals have the facility for the operator to override the AED and deliver a shock independently of any prompting by the machine.

The main advantages of AEDs are that they recognise specific shockable rhythms and therefore a shock can be delivered by a lay-person. They are also relatively cheap and lightweight and have therefore replaced many manual defibrillators. Available AEDs have been tested extensively against libraries of adult ECG rhythms and in trials in adults and children. They are extremely accurate in rhythm recognition in both adults and children. The voice prompts from the AED **must be followed** to ensure safe, effective practice.

If a child > 25 kg (approximately eight years) requires defibrillation, standard adult AED energy levels can be used.

If a child of < 25 kg (or eight years) requires emergency defibrillation, and there is no manual defibrillator available, an AED can be used. The AED should ideally be equipped with a dose attenuator, which decreases the delivered energy to a lower, more appropriate dosage (generally 50–75 J).

If such an AED is unavailable in an emergency situation, then a standard AED with adult energy levels may be used. The upper dose limit for safe defibrillation is unknown but higher doses than the previously recommended 4 J kg^{-1} have defibrillated children effectively and without significant adverse effects. Higher doses are acceptable because defibrillation is the only effective treatment for VF/pVT.

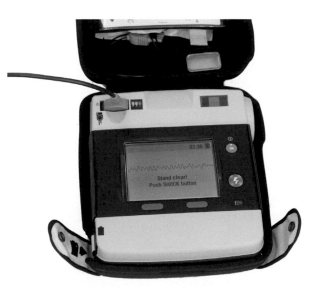

Figure 7.4 Automated external defibrillator (AED)

Infants have a much lower incidence of shockable rhythms and good quality CPR is the treatment priority. If an infant is in a shockable rhythm however and a manual machine is not available, use of an AED (preferably with attenuator) may be considered.

Minimal interruption to chest compression

Every time chest compressions are interrupted, even for a brief period, coronary and cerebral perfusion pressures fall and several compressions are needed to return these pressures to their previous levels. Interruptions should therefore be minimised during the defibrillation sequence.

- If a shockable rhythm is still present the manual defibrillator should be charged whilst chest compressions are continued.

- Compressions should be resumed straight after the shock with no check of either the monitor or patient.

Safety issues when undertaking defibrillation

The safety of the rescuers as well as that of the child is paramount. The following factors must be considered:

Oxygen

All free-flowing oxygen delivery devices (O_2 masks or nasal cannulae) must be removed from the immediate area and placed at least one metre from the child. If the child is being ventilated via a tracheal tube, the ventilation bag or ventilator tubing can be left connected if it forms part of a closed circuit. If the circuit is disconnected for whatever reason, the devices must be placed at least one metre away from the child.

Dry surfaces

Any wet clothing should be removed from the immediate area. The surface the child is laid on and the child's chest should be wiped dry if necessary, before shock delivery.

Contact with patient

The person delivering the shock must ensure that neither they nor any other rescuers/relatives are in direct or indirect contact with the child during shock delivery.

There should be no contact between the pads and any metal objects (e.g. jewellery) or items such as transdermal medication or diathermy pads.

Operator instructions

Familiarity with the defibrillator being used increases safety and operator efficiency. Operators must also ensure that they issue clear instructions to the rest of the team/bystanders to facilitate safe practice throughout the procedure.

Sequence of actions for manual asynchronous defibrillation

Having confirmed cardiorespiratory arrest, CPR should be started (or restarted) while the person delivering the shock prepares as follows:

1. Confirm presence of shockable rhythm (VF/pVT) via self-adhesive/monitoring pads or ECG monitor during brief pause in chest compressions.

2. Resume chest compressions immediately while designated person applies self-adhesive pads (if not already applied) on the child's chest.

3. The designated person selects the appropriate energy (4 J kg^{-1}) and presses the charge button.

4. While the defibrillator is charging warn all rescuers other than the individual performing the chest compressions to "stand clear", and remove any oxygen delivery device as appropriate.

5. Once the defibrillator is charged, tell the rescuer doing the chest compressions to "stand clear"; when clear and after confirming continued VF/pVT, give the shock.

6. Without reassessing the rhythm or feeling for a pulse, restart CPR starting with chest compressions.

7. Continue CPR for two minutes; the team leader prepares the team for the next pause in CPR (steps 3 and 4).

8. If VF/pVT persists deliver a second shock (as for steps 5 and 6).

Further management of shockable cardiac arrest rhythms is described in Chapter 8.

Considerations when using an AED

The AED pads are placed in the same position as manual defibrillators (Figure 7.1).

Sequence of actions for using an AED

The following guidance should be used for all AEDs, with or without a paediatric dose attenuating device:

1. Ensure safety of the child and rescuers/bystanders.

2. Start BLS. If more than one rescuer is available, one should summon help as appropriate, and then return to assist with BLS and attachment of the AED.

   If only one rescuer is available, they should perform one minute of CPR before going for help/collecting and attaching the AED (unless a cardiac cause is suspected).

3. Switch on the AED and attach self-adhesive pads. If more than one rescuer is present, BLS should be continued whilst the AED is attached.

4. Follow the AED prompts.

5. **Ensure no-one touches the child while the rhythm is being analysed.** This is extremely important as artefact from chest compressions given during analysis phase may be interpreted by the AED as VF and the machine may charge and advise a shock.

6. If defibrillation is indicated:

   - ensure no-one touches the child

   - press the shock delivery button as directed

   - continue as directed by the AED prompts.

7. If no shock is indicated:

   - resume BLS immediately

   - continue as directed by the AED prompts.

8. Continue resuscitation until:

   - help arrives and takes over management

   - the child starts to show 'signs of life'

   - the rescuer becomes too exhausted to continue.

NB Do not switch off the AED whilst CPR is continued.

Testing the defibrillator

Defibrillators should be regularly tested as per manufacturer and local policies. All potential operators should familiarise themselves with the specific operating procedures of their available machines.

Considerations when undertaking synchronised DC cardioversion

Cardioversion is the timed delivery of an electrical shock from the defibrillator. It is a procedure that can be used in the treatment of symptomatic SVT or VT with a pulse. The delivery of the electric shock is synchronised with the R wave of the ECG to minimise the risk of inducing VF.

The application of the pads and the safety precautions are the same as for asynchronous defibrillation, but there are some additional considerations. These include:

- Sedation/anaesthesia needs to be administered (if the child is conscious) before synchronised cardioversion is performed.

- Synchronisation mode on the defibrillator must be activated and on some machines it may need to be re-selected if repeat shock(s) are required or if the machine is accidentally turned off between shocks.

- Increase the ECG gain to ensure the defibrillator identifies all the R waves on the child's ECG.

- Energy levels for synchronised cardioversion are lower than for asynchronous defibrillation. The initial dose is 1 J kg^{-1} although this may be increased to 2 J kg^{-1} if the arrhythmia persists.

- ECG electrodes in addition to pads are needed for some defibrillators to operate in the synchronised mode.

- Delay in shock delivery can occur between the operator depressing the delivery button and the actual shock being delivered. This is because the machine will only deliver the shock when it identifies an R wave. In practice it means that the operator must keep the shock delivery button depressed until this occurs.

Following cardioversion, some defibrillators may remain in the synchronised mode which is a potential risk; a defibrillator left in the synchronised mode will not be immediately ready to deliver a shock to treat a VF/ pVT cardiorespiratory arrest victim, therefore always leave the defibrillator in the non-synchronised mode.

Summary learning

- **For the patient in VF/pVT, early defibrillation is the only effective means of restoring a spontaneous circulation.**

- **When using a defibrillator, minimise interruptions in chest compressions.**

- **Use an AED if you are not confident in rhythm recognition or manual defibrillation.**

My key take-home messages from this chapter

pILS

Management of cardiorespiratory arrest

Contents

- **Resuscitation process**
- **In-hospital cardiorespiratory arrest sequence**
- **Non-shockable rhythms**
- **Shockable rhythms**
- **Ongoing resuscitation**
- **Reversible causes of cardiorespiratory arrest**

Learning outcomes

To enable you to:
- **Plan for effective management of the resuscitation team**
- **Describe the importance of the team huddle**
- **Manage resuscitation until experienced help arrives**
- **Understand the importance of high quality cardiopulmonary resuscitation**
- **Identify the potentially reversible causes of cardiorespiratory arrest**
- **Consider when to stop resuscitation attempts**

Resuscitation process

The division between basic life support (BLS) and advanced life support (ALS) is somewhat artificial. Resuscitation is a continuous process, and the elements of effective BLS must be continued until return of a spontaneous circulation (ROSC), even when experienced help arrives (i.e. the EMS or clinical emergency team) and appropriate equipment can be used to facilitate delivery of advanced techniques. It is important that the on-call resuscitation team prepare for this event at changeover of staff and team huddles.

All clinical staff within a healthcare facility should be able to:

- immediately recognise cardiorespiratory arrest
- start appropriate resuscitation (BLS with available adjuncts)
- summon the clinical emergency team using the standard telephone number (2222 in-hospital) and/or EMS (via national 999 or 112 system)

The exact sequence of actions will be dependent on several factors including:
- location of event (clinical or non-clinical area)
- number of first responders
- skills of first responders
- availability of resuscitation equipment
- local policies.

Location of event

Clinical area

If the child is seriously ill on a ward, it is likely that they will have been deteriorating over a period of time. Many wards now employ an 'early warning scoring system' based on physiological parameters (e.g. paediatric early warning score (PEWS)), which is designed to identify seriously ill children before they become decompensated; experienced staff are alerted and can initiate appropriate management strategies to prevent cardiorespiratory arrest occurring.

When a child does suffer a cardiorespiratory arrest in a clinical area staff should be able to promptly initiate BLS and put out a 2222 call to summon the clinical emergency/cardiac arrest team. Appropriate resuscitation equipment and trained staff should be readily available.

Non-clinical area

There may be occasions when a child suffers a cardiorespiratory arrest in a non-clinical area (e.g. corridors, car park, play area). In these areas, there may not be readily available equipment or trained staff, and these children may have a more prolonged period of BLS before help arrives.

The guidance in this chapter is primarily aimed at healthcare professionals who may be an initial responder in a clinical emergency situation and have rapid access to resuscitation equipment.

Number of first responders

A single rescuer must not leave the collapsed child, but should start appropriate resuscitation (e.g. BLS or BLS with BMV) and ensure that further help is summoned. If the condition is thought to be due to a primary cardiac cause EMS help is activated before BLS has started. Within a clinical area, nearby staff can be alerted, either by the first responder shouting for help and/or using an emergency call button system. As soon as a second rescuer arrives, they should be sent to summon further assistance in line with local policy (i.e. activate the clinical emergency team by calling 2222). On their return (or the arrival of other staff) simultaneous interventions can be undertaken, according to the skills of the available staff.

Skills of first responders

Healthcare providers should be able to recognise cardiorespiratory arrest, shout for help and start resuscitation to the level to which they have been trained. The decay in resuscitation skills after training is well documented with skills retention probably lasting about 3 months. Recent studies indicate that short targeted refresher training for staff looking after the sicker patients at the bedside may be beneficial, so called 'just in time' training.

Staff will have been trained to different levels according to local policies; some may only undertake BLS, whilst others would be expected to undertake additional techniques to manage airway, breathing and circulation. First responders should only undertake the skills they have been trained to perform; their initial priority in paediatric cardiorespiratory arrest should be to ensure effective ventilation and oxygenation with good quality BLS. As more experienced help arrives, other interventions can be undertaken.

Availability of resuscitation equipment

All clinical areas where children are likely to be cared for should be equipped with resuscitation equipment to help with the management of a clinical emergency. The staff in each area should have responsibility for maintenance and regular checking of this clinical emergency equipment, as this will facilitate their familiarity with it. By employing standardised resuscitation equipment hospital-wide, the clinical emergency team should also know exactly what equipment is readily available to them when called to deal with a child in any area. Equipment capable of delivering CPR feedback for rescuers will improve the quality of CPR given and is advocated.

Local policies

As well as specifying the levels of resuscitation skills for different staff groups, hospitals should also have policies regarding the composition of, and calling criteria for, their clinical emergency teams. In some centres, there might be more than one emergency team (dictated by the geographical layout or the clinical specialties of the hospital) or there may be different types of team (e.g. a cardiac arrest team and a medical emergency team). Staff must be aware of their local systems and trained to act accordingly.

Cardiac arrest teams should meet at the beginning of each shift to introduce themselves to each other, discuss each team member's skills and assign roles. These 'huddles' will improve teamwork, particularly communication. Cardiac arrest teams will also operate more efficiently if their skills can be practised (and their effectiveness measured) by undertaking 'mock' emergency calls. This includes consideration of team organisation at a resuscitation event.

These operational issues should be audited. They can be practised (and their effectiveness measured) by undertaking 'mock' emergency calls.

In-hospital cardiorespiratory arrest sequence

The initial management of an apparently collapsed child is summarised in Figure 8.1.

Safety

The approach described in Chapter 3 should be followed to ensure firstly the safety of the rescuers and then that of the child. Whilst the risk of contracting infection is low, personal protective measures should be employed as soon as practicable (e.g. gloves, aprons, eye protection, face masks). In situations where the child may have a severe infection (e.g. open TB, Swine flu or SARS) rescuers must be equipped with full protective measures. In areas where such children may be treated, this equipment should be immediately available.

Stimulate

The approach described in Chapter 3 should be followed to establish the responsiveness of an apparently unconscious child.

Responsive child

If the child responds (i.e. they demonstrate 'signs of life'), the child should be assessed using an ABCDE approach.

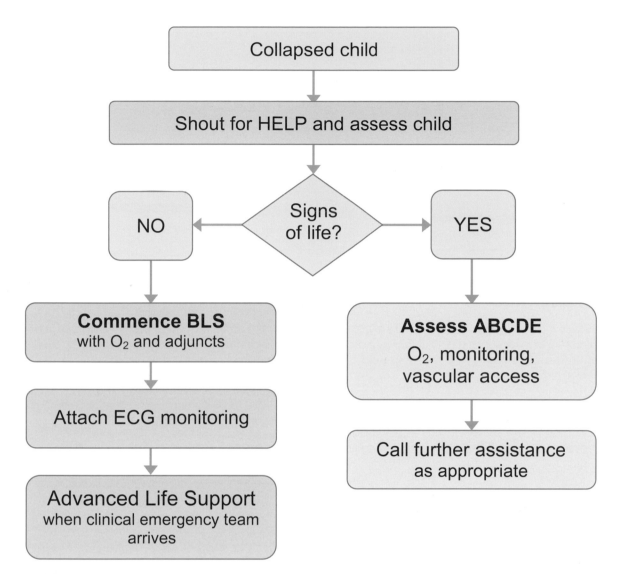

Figure 8.1 Initial resuscitation management

Appropriate interventions should be initiated and further relevant assistance summoned.

Unresponsive child

If the child is unresponsive (i.e. they do not demonstrate 'signs of life'), BLS must be started immediately whilst simultaneously shouting for more assistance.

Shout for help

The single rescuer must not leave the child but shout loudly for help and start BLS, using basic airway adjuncts and BMV if they are immediately available. It would also be appropriate for them to activate a bedside emergency call button system if this is available.

If there is a second rescuer available they should be sent to summon more assistance, and return to help with the resuscitation attempt. If there is resuscitation equipment nearby, they should bring this to the bedside, but this must not delay calling the clinical emergency team.

Airway

The airway should be opened as described in Chapter 3. If there is suction available, it may be necessary to use this to clear any secretions in the upper airway before proceeding to ventilation.

Breathing

If the child is not breathing, or only gasping ineffectively, initial rescue breaths should be delivered by the most appropriate method available (e.g. expired air rescue breaths with a barrier device or self-inflating bag-mask device with supplemental oxygen).

As soon as resuscitation equipment is available, the emphasis is on ensuring that effective CPR is enhanced by BMV with supplemental oxygen.

If there are two rescuers available and at least one is trained in the use of BMV, the rescuer managing the airway and delivering the rescue breaths should be positioned behind the child's head. A second rescuer should be positioned at the side of the child to perform chest compressions if indicated.

Circulation

Assessment

If a child, who is not breathing adequately, does not respond quickly to rescue breaths, they are unlikely to have an adequate spontaneous circulation. However, in the hospital setting, it is appropriate for a rescuer to briefly try and determine the presence of a central pulse whilst simultaneously observing for 'signs of life'.

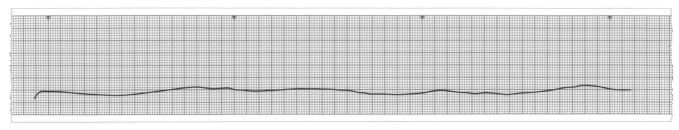

Figure 8.2 Asystole

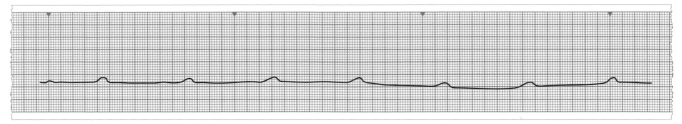

Figure 8.3 P-wave asystole

If an adequate pulse (i.e. > 60 min⁻¹) is DEFINITELY felt, but breathing is absent or inadequate, the child's airway must be maintained and rescue breathing continued at a rate of 12–20 min⁻¹.

If the child's pulse is absent or inadequate (i.e. < 60 min⁻¹), or there is any doubt and there are no other 'signs of life', chest compressions must be started. Ventilations and compressions are then delivered in 15:2 ratio until monitoring is attached.

Rhythm recognition

As soon as resuscitation equipment is available, the emphasis is on ensuring that effective CPR is enhanced by BMV with supplemental oxygen. The next step is to establish the child's cardiac rhythm, preferably with a defibrillator with CPR feedback capability. The priority is deciding whether the cardiac rhythm is shockable or not, in order to determine the ongoing management of the cardiorespiratory arrest. If an AED is used, the machine will guide the rescuers through the appropriate sequence of actions. However, in paediatric areas of a hospital, an ECG monitor, usually a manual defibrillator, is commonly available and therefore the clinical emergency team members must be able to rapidly identify whether they are dealing with a child in a shockable or nonshockable rhythm. Briefly pause chest compressions to allow for rhythm recognition on the monitor.

Shockable or non-shockable cardiac rhythms

In children, the most common initial cardiorespiratory arrest rhythms are non-shockable (i.e. profound bradycardia, asystole or pulseless electrical activity (PEA)).

The shockable cardiorespiratory arrest rhythms (i.e. ventricular fibrillation (VF) and pulseless ventricular tachycardia (pVT)) are less common. When these occur, it is often in a child with underlying cardiac disease.

The management of shockable and non-shockable cardiorespiratory arrest is outlined below.

Non-shockable rhythms (asystole and PEA)

Asystole

This rhythm is characterised by the total absence of effective electrical and mechanical activity in the heart (Figure 8.2).

It can be simulated by artefact (e.g. detached ECG leads/electrodes) so it is important to quickly check the equipment. In asystole, there is no ventricular function, but occasionally there is some residual atrial activity, which may be seen on the ECG as P waves (Figure 8.3). It is often preceded by severe bradycardia. The most common cause of bradycardia in a child is hypoxia.

Pulseless Electrical Activity (PEA)

This rhythm is defined as organised cardiac electrical activity in the absence of a palpable central pulse. It is thought that some of these children may have some myocardial contraction, but it is too weak and ineffective to produce a detectable pulse or blood pressure. The ECG rhythm displayed is often a slow, broad complex one, although any variation of regular QRS complexes may be seen.

All the cardiac arrest rhythms may be due to an underlying reversible condition (see below); it is essential that any treatable causes are identified and managed, these are listed within the paediatric advanced life support algorithm (Figure 8.4).

Management of asystole and PEA

- **Perform continuous CPR:**
  - Continue to ventilate with high-concentration oxygen.
  - If ventilating with bag-mask use a ratio of 15 chest compressions to 2 ventilations.
  - Use a compression rate of 100–120 min⁻¹. Depth approximately 4 cm in an infant, and 5cm in a child.
  - If the patient is intubated, chest compressions can be continuous as long as this does not interfere with satisfactory ventilation.
  - Once the child's trachea has been intubated and compressions are uninterrupted use a ventilation rate of approximately 10–12 min⁻¹. Note: once there is return of spontaneous circulation (ROSC), the ventilation rate should be 12–20 per min⁻¹. Measure end-tidal CO_2 to monitor ventilation and ensure correct tracheal tube placement.

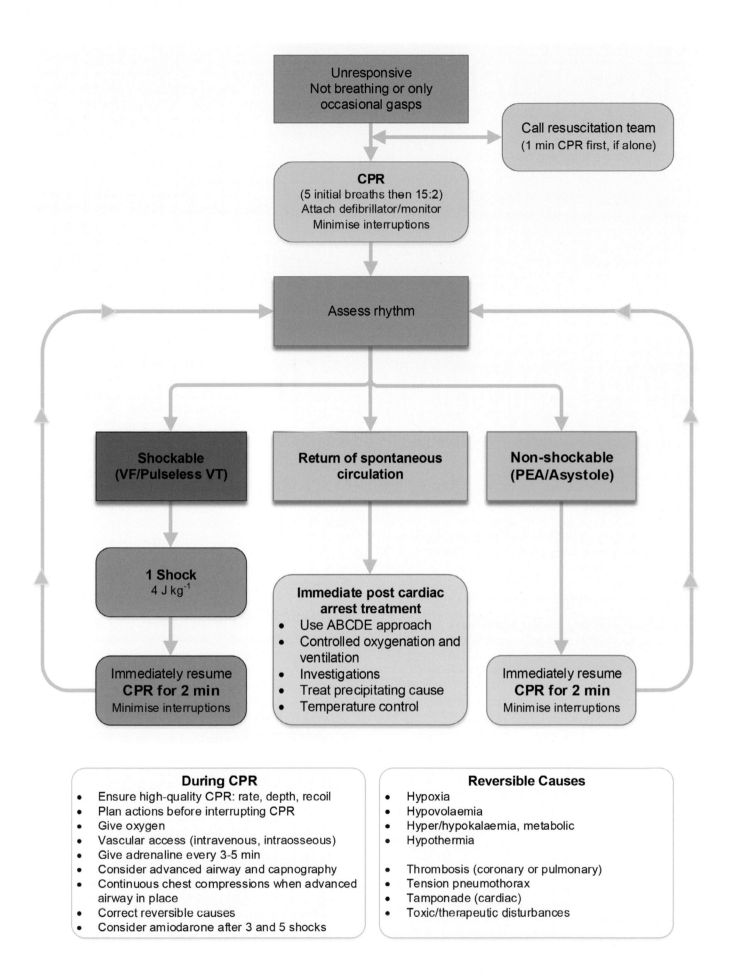

Figure 8.4 Paediatric advanced life support algorithm G2015

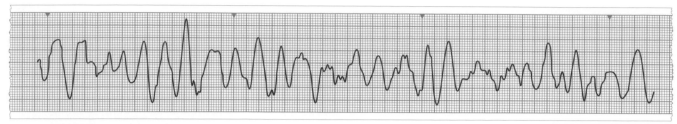

Figure 8.5 Coarse ventricular fibrillation

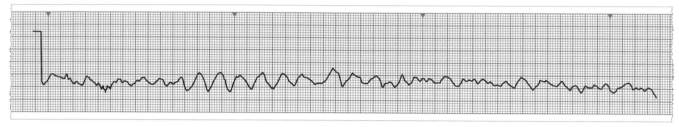

Figure 8.6 Fine ventricular fibrillation

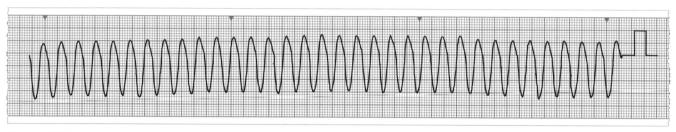

Figure 8.7 Ventricular tachycardia

- **Give adrenaline:**

  - If vascular access has been established, give adrenaline 10 mcg kg^{-1} (0.1 mL kg^{-1} of 1 in 10,000 solution).

  - If there is no circulatory access, obtain IO access

- **Continue CPR, only pausing briefly every 2 min to check for rhythm change**

  - Give adrenaline 10 mcg kg^{-1} every 3 to 5 min, (i.e. every other loop), while continuing to maintain effective chest compression and ventilation without interruption.

  - Good quality CPR is maximised if a feedback device is used.

- **Consider and correct reversible causes:** (4Hs and 4Ts)

- **If, during the rhythm check, organised electrical activity is seen on the monitor, check for 'signs of life' and a central pulse:**

  - If a pulse > 60 min^{-1} and/or 'signs of life' are present, start post resuscitation care.

  - If there is no pulse, or you are unsure, and there are no 'signs of life' (i.e. PEA) continue with 'non-shockable' algorithm.

If the cardiac rhythm changes to VF or pVT, the rescuers must change their management to follow the shockable side of the paediatric advanced life support algorithm (Figure 8.4).

Shockable rhythms (VF/pVT)

Ventricular fibrillation

This rhythm shows rapid, chaotic, irregular waves of varying frequency and amplitude. VF is sometimes classified as 'coarse or fine' depending on the amplitude (height) of the complexes (Figures 8.5 and 8.6). When there is doubt as to whether a rhythm is fine VF or asystole, rescuers should not deliver a defibrillation shock but should continue with CPR. It is unlikely that fine VF will be successfully shocked into a perfusing rhythm, but continuing good quality CPR may increase the frequency and amplitude of the VF and improve the chances of successful defibrillation (i.e. to produce a perfusing rhythm). If the cardiac rhythm is clearly VF, defibrillation should be performed without delay.

Pulseless VT (pVT)

This rhythm is a broad complex tachycardia (Figure 8.7). It is rare in children and is managed in the same way as VF (i.e. defibrillation).

Management of VF/pVT

- Continue CPR with BMV and supplemental O$_2$ until a defibrillator is available.

- **Defibrillate the heart:**

  o Charge the defibrillator while another rescuer continues chest compressions.

  o Once the defibrillator is charged, pause the chest compressions, quickly ensure that all rescuers are clear of the patient and then deliver the shock. This should be planned before stopping compressions.

  o Give 1 shock of 4 J kg^{-1} if using a manual defibrillator.

  o If using an AED for a child of less than 8 years, deliver a paediatric-attenuated adult shock energy.

  o If using an AED for a child over 8 years, use the adult shock energy.

- **Resume CPR:**

  o Without reassessing the rhythm or feeling for a pulse, resume CPR immediately, starting with chest compression.

  o Good quality CPR is maximised if a feedback device is used.

  o Consider and correct reversible causes (4Hs and 4Ts).

- **Continue CPR for 2 min, then pause briefly to check the monitor:**

  o If still VF/pVT, give a second shock (with same energy level and strategy for delivery as the first shock).

  - **Resume CPR:**

    o Without reassessing the rhythm or feeling for a pulse, resume CPR immediately, starting with chest compression.

- **Continue CPR for 2 min, then pause briefly to check the monitor:**

- **If still VF/pVT, give a third shock** (with same energy level and strategy for delivery as the previous shock).

  - **Resume CPR:**

    o Without reassessing the rhythm or feeling for a pulse, resume CPR immediately, starting with chest compression.

    o Give adrenaline 10 mcg kg^{-1} and amiodarone 5 mg kg^{-1} after the third shock, once chest compressions have resumed.

    o Repeat adrenaline every alternate cycle (i.e. every 3–5 min) until ROSC.

    o Repeat amiodarone 5 mg kg^{-1} one further time, after the fifth shock if still in a shockable rhythm.

- Continue giving shocks every 2 min, continuing compressions during charging of the defibrillator and minimising the breaks in chest compression as much as possible.

  o **After each 2 min of uninterrupted CPR, pause briefly to assess the rhythm: If still VF/pVT:**

    ▪ Continue CPR with the shockable (VF/pVT) sequence.

  o **If asystole:**

    ▪ Continue CPR and switch to the non-shockable (asystole or PEA) sequence as above.

  o **If organised electrical activity is seen,** check for signs of life and a pulse:

    ▪ If there is ROSC, continue post-resuscitation care.

    ▪ If there is no pulse (or a pulse rate of <60 min^{-1}), and there are no other signs of life, continue CPR and continue as for the non-shockable sequence above.

- If defibrillation was successful but VF/pVT recurs, resume the CPR sequence and defibrillate. Give an amiodarone bolus (unless two doses have already been given) and start a continuous infusion of the drug.

Important note

Uninterrupted, high quality CPR is vital. Chest compression and ventilation should be interrupted only for defibrillation. Chest compression is tiring for providers and the team leader should repeatedly assess and feedback on the quality of the compressions. To prevent fatigue, change providers should every two minutes. This will mean that the team can deliver effective high quality CPR so improving the chances of survival.

Rationale for sequence of actions on shockable side of algorithm

- The interval between stopping chest compressions and delivering a shock must be minimal (< 10 s); longer interruptions to chest compressions reduce the likelihood of a shock restoring a perfusing rhythm.

- Chest compressions are resumed immediately after a shock without reassessing the rhythm or feeling for a pulse because, even if the defibrillation attempt is successful in restoring a rhythm, it is unlikely that the heart will immediately pump effectively. Even if a perfusing rhythm has been restored, giving chest compressions does not increase the chance of VF recurring

If an organised rhythm is observed during a 2 min cycle of CPR, **do not interrupt chest compressions to palpate a pulse, unless the patient shows signs of life** demonstrating return of spontaneous circulation (ROSC).

If there is any doubt about the presence of a pulse in a patient who has an organised cardiac rhythm compatible with cardiac output, but no other signs of life, resume CPR for a further 2 min.

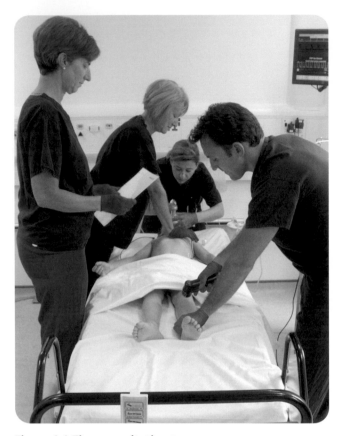

Figure 8.8 The resuscitation team

Ongoing resuscitation

Outcome in all resuscitation attempts is dependent on good quality chest compressions and ventilation (plus defibrillation when indicated for shockable arrhythmias). Performing chest compression is tiring, and to reduce fatigue and maximise efficiency, the rescuer delivering chest compressions should share the work with another by alternating at least every 2 min. As soon as the airway is secured with a tracheal tube, chest compressions should be performed continuously unless this compromises delivery of adequate tidal volumes.

Airway and ventilation

The vast majority of children can be adequately ventilated with BMV in the initial stages of resuscitation; it is often better to continue with this until ROSC rather than attempt tracheal intubation and temporarily interrupt oxygenation during laryngoscopy. However, once the expertise is available, tracheal intubation provides the most reliable airway and will be essential in the post-resuscitation management of a child who has suffered cardiorespiratory arrest.

If laryngoscopy is to be performed during CPR, it should be attempted without interruption of chest compressions, although there may need to be a brief pause as the

tracheal tube is passed through the vocal cords. Following tracheal intubation and confirmation of the correct tube position, the tube should be secured, capnography attached and then chest compressions can be delivered continuously without a pause for ventilation. Breaths should be delivered at a rate of approximately 10–12 min⁻¹.

Circulatory access

If the child does not already have secure circulatory access, this should be achieved as soon as possible after establishing effective CPR during a cardiorespiratory arrest. The emergency route of choice is intraosseous (IO).

History and reversible causes

Obtaining relevant information about the child's underlying medical condition and any pre-disposing events can be useful in determining likely causes of, and potential outcome from, the cardiorespiratory arrest.

Any possible causes (or aggravating factors) that have specific treatment must be considered during all cardiorespiratory arrests. The most likely of these can be recalled by the mnemonic '4 Hs and 4 Ts':

The 4 Hs

1. **Hypoxia**
2. **Hypovolaemia**
3. **Hypo/hyperkalaemia/metabolic**
4. **Hypothermia**

The 4 Ts

1. **Tension pneumothorax**
2. **Tamponade (cardiac)**
3. **Toxins/therapeutic disturbance**
4. **Thrombosis (coronary or pulmonary)**

Hypoxia

This is a frequent cause of paediatric cardiorespiratory arrest. The risks of it occurring, or persisting, during resuscitation should be minimised by ensuring effective ventilation with 100% oxygen. It is essential to ensure that there is adequate, bilateral chest movement. The mnemonic DOPES described in Chapter 9 should be considered in intubated children.

Hypovolaemia

Loss of circulating volume can often result in cardiorespiratory arrest. When a child shows signs of circulatory failure, controlled volume administration is indicated. Hypovolaemia may be due to many different causes (e.g. haemorrhage from trauma, diarrhoea and vomiting, anaphylaxis, severe sepsis) and these need to be identified and treated appropriately. If signs of circulatory failure are present, start rapid circulatory volume replacement with an initial bolus of 20 mL kg^{-1} of 0.9% saline solution; volume and frequency of bolus is discussed in Chapter 5.

Hypo/hyperkalaemia, metabolic

Electrolyte and metabolic disorders may be suggested by the child's medical history and/or biochemical tests. Specific treatment should be given to correct these problems. An estimation of blood glucose level should be obtained early; both hypo and hyperglycaemia are common and associated with increased morbidity and mortality.

Hypothermia

Low body temperature may be an unlikely problem in hospitalised children, but it should always be considered, particularly in small or premature infants, or in children being managed in the emergency department. A low-reading thermometer should be used to record a core temperature when hypothermia is considered a possibility.

Tension pneumothorax

Signs of tension pneumothorax (e.g. decreased chest movement and air entry, hyper-resonance on the affected side, tracheal deviation away from the affected side) should be sought, particularly in children who have suffered trauma, following thoracic surgery or who have an acute asthmatic attack. If a tension pneumothorax is thought to be present, rapid needle decompression is required, followed by chest drain insertion.

Tamponade (cardiac)

This is not a common cause of cardiorespiratory arrest in children, but may occur following cardiothoracic surgery, penetrating chest trauma or some viral illnesses. It can be difficult to diagnose as typical signs (e.g. distended neck veins and hypovolaemia) are often masked by the cardiorespiratory arrest. If there is a strong history, needle pericardiocentesis is indicated.

Toxins/therapeutic disturbances

In the absence of a confirmed history, accidental or deliberate poisoning with toxins (therapeutic or toxic substances) may only be discovered after laboratory analysis. Appropriate antidotes should be administered as soon as possible when indicated and available, but frequently management of these children is based on measures to support their vital organs. Check the patient's drug chart.

Thrombosis (coronary or pulmonary)

It is unusual for children to suffer from thromboembolic complications, but they can occur. If it is considered that this is a cause, appropriate thrombolysis would be needed.

Stopping resuscitation

Resuscitation efforts are less likely to be successful in achieving ROSC if there have been no signs of cardiac output, despite at least 20–30 min of continuous, good quality CPR in children. However, occasionally good quality survival has been reported for longer durations of CPR, so the circumstances of the cardiac arrest, the age and the presenting rhythm must all be taken into consideration when making the decision to stop resuscitation; CPR is more often successful in children > 1 year of age and in those presenting with VF or pVT.

However, it would be appropriate to prolong resuscitation attempts in children with the following conditions:

- hypothermia
- poisoning
- persistent VF/pVT.

The resuscitation team may also consider that specific circumstances (e.g. awaiting arrival of family members) make it appropriate to maintain resuscitation efforts.

Presence of parents during resuscitation

The opportunity to be present during at least part of the resuscitation of their child should be offered to parents/carers. Evidence suggests that this aids with their grieving process (less anxiety and depression when assessed several months later).

The following points (which apply whether the parent is actually in the room beside their child, or elsewhere in the ward/department) should be considered:

- A specific member of staff should be delegated to remain with the parents throughout to offer empathetic, but realistic, support.

- If necessary, an appropriate interpreter must be present to facilitate accuracy of communication between parents and the resuscitation team leader.

- Physical contact with their child and the opportunity to say 'goodbye' (in unsuccessful resuscitation attempts) should be encouraged.

- The resuscitation team leader decides when to stop resuscitation efforts, and not the parents.

- A debriefing session for all staff involved should be arranged to offer support and reflect on practice.

- Appropriate referrals and counselling should be organised for the parents to ensure they receive adequate support.

Summary learning

- The optimal management of in-hospital cardiorespiratory arrest is always based on the rapid initiation of effective ventilation, oxygenation and chest compression.

- The paediatric advanced life support algorithm provides a framework for cardiorespiratory arrest management of all children.

- Asystole and PEA are non-shockable arrhythmias and their management is based on effective CPR, adrenaline administration and treatment of reversible causes.

- VF and pVT are shockable arrhythmias and their management is based on effective CPR, early defibrillation and treatment of reversible causes.

- The parents/carers should be supported and, ideally, be present during the resuscitation of their child.

My key take-home messages from this chapter

Post-resuscitation care, stabilisation and transfer

Chapter 9

Contents

- Post cardiac arrest syndrome pathology and management
- Preventing secondary injury via ABCDE assessment and management
- Preparing for transfer/retrieval of children to other facilities for ongoing care

Learning outcomes

To enable you to:

- **Understand the importance of post-resuscitation stabilisation and optimisation of organ function following cardiorespiratory arrest**
- **Describe the specific investigations and monitoring indicated**
- **Facilitate the safe transfer of the seriously ill child**

Continued resuscitation

Cardiorespiratory arrest represents the most severe shock state during which delivery of oxygen and metabolic substrates to tissues is abruptly halted. Cardiopulmonary resuscitation (CPR) only partially reverses this process, achieving cardiac output and systemic oxygen delivery that is much less than normal. The aim is to restore oxygenation and perfusion to the vital organs as rapidly as possible to minimise the primary injury. For children who have had a cardiorespiratory arrest the initial step is restoration of spontaneous circulation (ROSC) but this is only the first step in the continuous process of resuscitation management. A significant percentage of resuscitated children ultimately die or survive with serious neurological sequelae so good post-resuscitation care is required to maintain organ perfusion and prevent secondary organ injury whenever possible.

Secondary organ damage includes:

- hypoxic-ischaemic brain injury
- ischaemic myocardial damage
- hypoxic pulmonary damage
- acute renal failure
- coagulopathy
- ischaemic hepatitis
- acute gastro-intestinal lesions.

The ABCDE approach must be followed in the immediate post-resuscitation phase as it focuses management priorities. However, the ongoing care of the child requires the expertise of many healthcare professionals and is best delivered in a paediatric intensive care (PICU) facility. This may require a specialist team to facilitate an optimal safe transfer.

pILS

Stabilisation of airway and breathing

The aim of respiratory management is to maintain adequate oxygenation and ventilation, avoiding hypoxia, hyperoxia and hypo/hypercapnia, which may worsen the child's prognosis.

If the child (or infant) has been resuscitated using BMV a decision needs to be made whether he will need ongoing ventilation and placement of a tracheal tube. Factors that may affect this decision include:

- conscious level (AVPU) at level P or less means that there will be no protective airway reflexes

- requirement for the safe transfer to a PICU

- lung pathology resulting in a need for respiratory support.

BMV causes gastric distention which will impede ventilation and may cause vomiting. A gastric tube is usually required to deflate the stomach if it has become distended following BMV.

Children and infants who remain intubated and ventilated will need sedation and analgesia in most cases.

Following intubation, the most common post-resuscitation airway/breathing complications can be identified by considering the acronym DOPES (Table 9.1).

Table 9.1 Possible airway and breathing complications following tracheal intubation

D	Displacement of tracheal tube (e.g. oesophagus, right main stem bronchus)
O	Obstruction of artificial airway (accumulated secretions, kinking)
P	Pneumothorax (from excessive BMV pressure, rib fractures)
E	Equipment failure (e.g. disconnected oxygen supply)
S	Stomach distension (following expired air or bag-mask ventilation)

Vital signs, such as blood gases and SpO_2 must be monitored post-resuscitation.

SpO_2 should be monitored continuously with a pulse oximeter and blood gas analysis should be performed as soon as possible. Although 100% oxygen is used for resuscitation, prolonged administration of high oxygen concentrations can result in pulmonary and cerebral toxicity. Once the child is stable, inspired oxygen should be gradually reduced to achieve an SpO_2 of between 94–98%.

End-tidal CO_2 monitoring is essential. This will confirm the correct location of a tracheal tube, allow continuous CO_2 monitoring during transport and support the optimisation of ventilation to maintain normocapnia. A chest X-ray should be obtained to identify lung pathology, check for rib fractures (very rare in children) and confirm the correct tracheal and gastric tube positions (Figure 9.1).

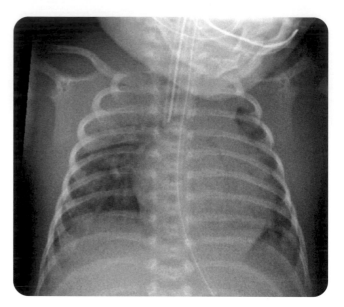

Figure 9.1 Chest X-ray showing tracheal tube at low position, causing right upper lobe collapse – this resolves when the tube is gently pulled back up the trachea.

If a resuscitated child has a tracheal tube in place and starts to make respiratory effort but remains unconscious, it is usually preferable to leave them intubated and ventilated (with appropriate sedation and analgesia) until after transfer and admission to PICU, since they can deteriorate rapidly, and reintubation during transfer is extremely hazardous.

Circulation

The aim of circulatory management is to ensure adequate organ perfusion and tissue oxygenation.

Haemodynamic function and cardiac rhythm are likely to be unstable in the immediate post-resuscitation phase but every effort should be made to try to optimise cardiac output and maintain blood pressure in the normal range. In addition to continuous ECG, SpO_2, end-tidal CO_2 and BP monitoring, vital organ perfusion should be assessed by recording urine output and peripheral perfusion (CRT and skin temperature) as a minimum. Ideally capillary refill time (CRT) should be < 2 s and the heart rate, blood pressure and respiratory rate should all be maintained within the age-appropriate range.

Systolic and mean BP are indirect measures of organ perfusion and can be obtained either non-invasively or continuously via an arterial line, (particularly useful for ventilated patients). Urine output should be > 1mL kg^{-1} h^{-1} in children. Assessment of central venous pressure (CVP), a measure of preload (i.e. the filling volume of the heart) may also be appropriate in some children but will require insertion of a central line. After fluid resuscitation palpation of the liver edge may also give an indication of fluid status (particularly in infants) and should normally be < 1 cm beyond the costal margin.

Assessment of the child's fluid balance and circulating volume must be considered. Resuscitation boluses of isotonic saline solutions, such as 0.9% saline or Hartmann's solution may be required to optimise circulating volume. Crystalloids can be safely used in the peri-resuscitation period but some patients may require blood or other colloids.

Maintenance fluids should be based on biochemistry evaluations and blood glucose should be measured. Glucose should be administered judiciously as required to avoid hypoglycaemia or hyperglycaemia as both conditions can have a deleterious effect on neurological outcome in critically unwell children. Careful monitoring is required. During the immediate post-resuscitation period, decisions about securing longer-term vascular access will be required (e.g. insertion of central venous cannulae to replace intraosseous access or additional lines to deliver specific medications).

Ongoing resuscitation of the child may necessitate inotrope infusions. These are preferably administered via dedicated central venous catheters. Having a central line with multiple lumens ensures that inotropes are not interrupted to deliver other medications and fluids, and avoids incompatibilities.

Disability

The brain is highly vulnerable to hypoxia and ischaemia. It can be injured by direct trauma, infection, hyper/hypoglycaemia, hypocapnia, seizures or raised intracranial pressure. Secondary brain injury can be minimised by stabilising systemic blood pressure, treating seizures, normalising blood gases (taking particular care to avoid hypoxia), correcting glucose and electrolyte abnormalities and actively preventing fever (normothermia must be aggressively maintained). The successfully resuscitated child with hypothermia and ROSC should not be immediately rewarmed actively unless the temperature is less than 32°C.

An assessment of neurological status should be performed early to obtain a post-resuscitation baseline, help identify neurological deficits and possibly help to predict prognosis.

Conscious level should be assessed with either the AVPU or Glasgow Coma Scale scoring systems. Pupil reactivity, posturing and focal signs should also be noted and regularly recorded.

Neuroprotective care post-ROSC aims to avoid secondary brain injury and should start from the first minutes after ROSC.

Exposure

Exposure and a full examination to detect any lesions (e.g. rashes, wounds) should be undertaken and may help in making the diagnosis, informing specific management of the child (e.g. the purpuric rash of meningococcaemia may prompt treatment with broad spectrum antibiotics if not already given). Care should be taken to respect the child's dignity and excessive hypothermia avoided especially in infants.

Other organs

Renal function should be monitored by measuring urine output, and the serum urea and creatinine levels. Insertion of a urinary catheter may be necessary. Treatment is directed towards maintaining an adequate circulating volume, which sustains renal perfusion. Hence diuretics are only indicated if decreased urine output persists after adequate fluid resuscitation. The gastrointestinal mucosa and liver can also be affected by hypoxia and ischaemia. Gastrointestinal mucosal injury can contribute to multi-organ failure, due to leakage of toxins and bacteria into the circulation. Treatment is aimed at maintaining adequate circulating volume and gut perfusion.

Further assessment

History

A comprehensive history is important to determine the cause of cardiorespiratory arrest, and plan ongoing management. This should include relevant details about the past medical history, previous health/ill health and medications, as well as precipitating events. Details about the initial management of the current event (e.g. delay in starting resuscitation) should also be sought, as these may influence ongoing management.

Investigations

The child's physiological parameters are likely to be deranged in the immediate post-resuscitation period; urgent haematological, biochemical, radiological and cardiological investigations may all be indicated (Table 9.2).

Facilitating safe patient transfer

Following cardiorespiratory stabilisation, the child should be safely transferred to an appropriate (PICU) for definitive and ongoing medical support. The decision to transfer should be made only after discussion between senior members of the PICU team, the clinical emergency team leader and the child's primary team (if available for consultation). Other considerations pre-transfer are listed in Table 9.3.

Table 9.2: Post-resuscitation investigations

Investigation	Rationale
Arterial blood gas (plus lactate)	• Ensure adequate ventilation • Assess tissue perfusion
Biochemistry	• Assess renal function • Maintain normoglycaemia • Assess electrolyte balance (especially Na^+, K^+, Mg^{2+}, Ca^+) • Liver function tests to look for ischaemic injury
Full blood count Clotting screen Group and Save	• Assess haemoglobin level and exclude anaemia • Monitor infection markers (e.g. white cell count, CRP etc) • Identify underlying blood disorders • Assess any coagulopathy from sepsis or ischaemia • Allows for urgent crossmatch
Chest X-ray	• Establish position of tracheal tube, central venous lines, gastric tube (as appropriate) • Detect underlying pathology (primary respiratory or cardiac disease, aspiration) • Exclude pneumothorax/rib fractures • Establish heart size

Other investigations as indicated (e.g. head CT or pelvis X-rays, cardiac echography, 12-lead ECG, serum and urine toxicology)

Table 9.3: Pre-transfer considerations

- Stabilise the child (ongoing or recurrent cardiorespiratory arrest precludes transfer).
- Arrange the most appropriate mode of transport.
- Inform the paediatric consultant and any other specialty lead involved in the immediate care of the child (e.g. anaesthetist, surgeon, department nurse in charge, child protection lead if appropriate).
- Inform child's parents of transfer details and ensure they have appropriate means of transport to the PICU.
- A. Ensure a secure airway (aspirate any endotracheal tube secretions prior to transfer).
- B. Ensure appropriate settings on transport ventilator, adequate portable oxygen supplies for length of journey, and alternative means of ventilating the child (manual ventilation circuit that can be used either with or without oxygen supply). Deflate stomach with passage of a gastric tube.
- C. Ensure adequate intravenous access.
- D. Ensure adequate sedation and analgesia being delivered +/- muscle relaxant and that sufficient drugs are available for the journey. Reassess pupillary reaction and conscious level.
- E. Ensure heat loss during transfer is kept to a minimum (unless intentionally cooling the patient) with insulation blankets and warming devices.
- F. Fluids: Ensure maintenance fluids are running and blood glucose levels are monitored. Consider a urinary catheter prior to transfer. Monitor urine output. Transfer all medication/fluid infusions and monitoring to portable transport devices.
- Contact PICU to update them of child's clinical status and provide estimated time of arrival before departure.
- Prepare full and clear records of the event including all interventions (copies of notes, drug charts, X-rays is ideal).
- Just prior to moving the child run through the ABCDE assessment aloud with all team members involved. Request any suggestions or comments from the team and then confirm with all team members that they are in agreement to move the patient.

Summary learning

- ROSC following cardiopulmonary resuscitation is merely the first step in the continuous process of resuscitation management.

- The ongoing management of seriously ill children includes appropriate vital sign monitoring, supportive therapies based on continuous ABCDE assessment and safe transfer to a PICU facility.

My key take-home messages from this chapter

pILS

Non-technical skills in resuscitation

Contents

- **Non-technical skills**
- **Situational awareness**
- **Decision making**
- **Team working including leadership**
- **Task management**
- **Resuscitation audit**

Learning outcomes

To enable you to:

- **Understand the role of non-technical skills in resuscitation**
- **Discuss the roles of team leader and team member**
- **Appreciate the importance of communication tools such as SBAR and RSVP for both summoning help and for handover**

Non technical skills

Paediatric resuscitation is particularly emotive and stressful and highly time critical. Outcomes can be improved by forward planning and practising teamwork skills and communication. The resuscitation team may take the form of a traditional cardiac arrest team, which is called only when cardiorespiratory arrest is recognised. However, many hospitals now have medical emergency teams who can manage sick children at risk of cardiorespiratory arrest and facilitate effective treatment thereby preventing it. The term 'resuscitation team' in this manual reflects the range of response teams.

Recently, the importance of team "huddles" has been recognised. This allows on-call staff to meet before shift changes/handovers, introduce each other and decide on role allocation. This 'huddle' prepares the team, maximises the team's ability to work closely and focus on the best care for the patient. After an emergency it is equally important to reflect on and scrutinise every aspect of the resuscitation from response times through to team actions and communication in order to identify areas for improvement.

Traditionally, advanced life support courses have focused mainly on skills: chest compressions, defibrillation, rhythm recognition and vascular access and the knowledge required to deliver optimal care. There is now a paradigm shift stressing the importance of many non-technical skills including communication, leadership, mutual support from team members, task distribution and situational awareness, leading to better decision making.

Deficiencies in the requisite non-technical skills are a common cause of adverse incidents.

Such deficiencies include:

- errors calling the resuscitation team
- failure to start CPR
- late or non arrival of personnel
- lack of organised cooperation in resuscitation teams
- lack of leadership
- poor communication.

Non-technical skills describe communication, situational awareness, decision-making, team working including leadership and task management.

Communication

- Communication problems are a factor in up to 80% of adverse incidents or near-miss reports in hospitals.
- Communication is vital in every stage of managing a sick child: summoning help, preparing for the resuscitation, during the resuscitation and organising the post resuscitation care.
- The use of the SBAR (Situation-Background-Assessment-Recommendation) or RSVP (Reason-Story-Vital signs-Plan) tool enables effective, timely communication between individuals from different clinical backgrounds and hierarchies and this can apply to both summoning help and performing a handover (Table 10.1). Clear unambiguous communication is essential to ensure that help arrives, information is handed over in a clear fashion, likely to be understood quickly and facilitating incorporation of a new team leader or team member.

Example of good communication:

A nurse finding a patient asks her colleague to call the resuscitation team.

"John, this child is in cardiorespiratory arrest, please dial 2222 and call the resuscitation team. Come back immediately with BMV when you have made the call."

Preparation

Responsibilities of a team leader on a shift:

Pre-planning during the 'huddle' helps the team identify a team leader (TL) and allocate tasks to different team members (TM) appropriately according to skill mix, identifying any immediate need for further senior help. Depending upon the number of team members the TL will assign tasks, as follows:

1. Airway and ventilation tasks.
2. Pulse check and chest compressions (alternate for chest compressions and recording/drug preparation).
3. Attaching monitoring, pads and/or defibrillating as indicated.

4. Gaining IO/IV access, preparing and delivering drugs.
5. Recording events, drug preparation.

Relatives can be looked after by another member of staff. This should not be the most junior member of staff as parents need careful explanation of the events .

After 2 min rescuers doing chest compressions become less effective so this task should be rotated with other team members. The TL can ask other team members to alternate if more appropriate. Ideally this change should be pre-planned and communicated to the rest of the team.

Clinical staff who participate as members of the resuscitation team must be up to date with advanced skills in paediatric life support, including resuscitation algorithms. They must be familiar and practised with local equipment such as the defibrillator, type of intra-osseous needles and auto-injectors.

It is also important that resuscitation teams practise skills together to try to avoid error through non-technical skills. This may involve high and low-fidelity scenarios on courses such as PILS and involve on-site mock clinical emergency team calls locally.

Management of the resuscitation

Some preparation can be made if there is time by writing up predicted weight, airway size, fluid and drug requirement, if the age or weight of the child is known. Remember, exact weight estimation is not necessary as most resuscitation drugs are based on lean weight.

- During the resuscitation phase, clear commands addressed directly to individuals keep a team focused and a team leader should use 'closed loop' techniques to ensure a task has been performed (e.g. "bloods taken, including gases and cross match 4 units packed cells").
- It may be helpful to ask in turn the findings of the team member dealing with the airway, then breathing and then the circulation, addressing any problems that are found as they are identified.

Situational awareness

This can be described as an individual's awareness of the environment at any one moment in a crisis and their ability to respond. How individuals react may impact on future events, this becomes particularly important when many events are happening simultaneously (e.g. at a cardiorespiratory arrest). High information input with poor situational awareness may result in poor decisions being made and poor quality CPR (for example, long gaps in chest compressions).

SBAR	RSVP	Content	Example
SITUATION	**R**EASON	• Introduce yourself and check you are speaking to the correct person • Identify the patient you are calling about (who and where) • Say what you think the current problem is, or appears to be • State what you need advice about • Useful phrases: - The problem appears to be cardiac/respiratory/neurological/sepsis - I'm not sure what the problem is but the patient is deteriorating - The patient is unstable, getting worse and I need help	• Hi, I'm Dr Smith the paediatric F2 • I am calling about Sam Brown on the paediatric ward who I think has a severe pneumonia and is septic • He has an oxygen saturation of 90% despite high-flow oxygen and I am very worried about him
BACKGROUND	**S**TORY	• Background information about the patient • Reason for admission • Relevant past medical history	• He is 6 years old and previously fit and well • He has had fever and a cough for 2 days • He was admitted yesterday
ASSESSMENT	**V**ITAL SIGNS	• Include specific observations and vital sign values based on ABCDE approach • Airway • Breathing • Circulation • Disability • Exposure • The early warning score is...	• He looks very unwell and is tiring • Airway – he can say a few words • Breathing – his respiratory rate is 34, he has widespread wheeze in both lung fields and has bronchial breathing on the left side. His oxygen saturation is 90% on high-flow oxygen. I am getting a blood gas and chest X-ray • Circulation – his pulse is 180, his blood pressure is 90/60 • Disability – he is drowsy and is clinging onto his mum • Exposure – he has no rashes
RECOMMENDATION	**P**LAN	• State explicitly what you want the person you are calling to do • What by when? • Useful phrases: - I am going to start the following treatment; is there anything else you can suggest? - I am going to do the following investigations; is there anything else you can suggest? - If they do not improve; when would you like to be called? - I don't think I can do any more; I would like you to see the patient urgently	• He is only on oral antibiotics so I am starting an IV • I need help – please can you come and see him straight away?

Table 10.1 SBAR and RSVP communication tools

At a cardiorespiratory arrest, all those participating will have varying degrees of situational awareness. In a well-functioning team, the team leader ensures all members will have a common understanding of current events, or shared situational awareness. This may be done by the team leader intermittently succinctly summing-up the situation, actions taken so far and planned actions, giving time for team members to provide any additional information or comment as appropriate. It is important that only the relevant information is shared.

Important situational awareness factors include:

- consideration of the location of the arrest, which can give clues to the cause

- obtaining information from staff about the events leading up to the arrest

- confirmation of the diagnosis if known or keeping track of tests ordered

- noting actions already initiated (e.g. chest compressions)

- checking that a monitor been attached and interpreting the rhythm

- gathering information from team members

- implementing any immediate necessary action and consideration of the likely impact of interventions

- determining the immediate needs

- not losing awareness of the overall situation when encountering difficult to overcome problems.

Decision making

This is defined as the cognitive process of choosing a specific course of action from several alternatives. At a cardiorespiratory arrest, decision making usually falls to the team leader who may be a nurse or junior doctor. The leader needs to establish their role quickly if not pre-planned, and assimilate information from those present to determine appropriate interventions. Typical decisions made include:

- confirmation of cardiorespiratory arrest and continuation of CPR

- attaching a monitor and assessing the rhythm

- delivering a shock if indicated

- considering the likely causes of the cardiac arrest.

Team working, including team leadership

A team is a group of people collaborating, cooperating and coordinating their activities towards a common goal. Team leadership can be taught, observed and practised. Team membership can be improved by rehearsal, reflection and coaching producing effective teams which lead them to perform well together.

Team leadership

The management of a sick child requires a team leader who communicates clearly providing guidance, direction, instruction and an overall update to the team members. Team leaders are facilitators, leading by example and integrity, and need experience, not simply seniority. Team leadership is achieved as a process, thereby it can become available to everyone with training and it is not restricted to those with leadership traits. There are several attributes recognisable in good team leaders:

- Ideally, the team leader knows everyone in the team by name and knows their capability.

- Accepts the leadership role and announces it early preferably at start of shift huddle so it is clear who is leading the team; this is very important as many people are reluctant to 'step up' and precious time is lost. The leader does need to be assertive and authoritative when appropriate and both knowledgeable and credible to influence the team through role modelling and professionalism.

- Is able to delegate tasks appropriately.

- The team leader should update the team, keeping them in the 'big picture' and should help include late additions to the team. This enables team members to offer constructive ideas/solutions or to challenge possible erroneous decisions. A leader will follow current resuscitation guidelines or explain the reasoning for any significant deviation from standard protocols. If a leader is unsure of a diagnosis or how to proceed then he or she should consult with the team or call for senior advice and assistance if appropriate.

- Remains calm and keeps everyone focused and controls distractions.

- Is a good communicator – not just good at giving instructions, also a good listener and decisive in action. A good leader also shows tolerance towards hesitancy or nervousness in the emergency setting, showing empathy towards the whole team.

- Allow the team autonomy if their skills are adequate (e.g. the anaesthetist may be delegated to be responsible for the airway management so 'leadership' of the airway is the anaesthetist's responsibility). When the airway is secured the anaesthetist should inform the team leader.

- Use the two-minute periods of chest compressions to prioritise and plan tasks and safety aspects of the resuscitation attempt with the team. If a case is particularly complex it may be necessary for the leadership style to change from facilitative to directive in order to drive the speed of treatment in the time critical situation.

- The team leader needs to watch for fatigue, stress and distress amongst the team and manage conflict.

- At the end of the resuscitation attempt, the leader should thank the team and ensure that staff and relatives are being supported and kept fully informed. Complete all documentation and ensure an adequate handover by planned communication with experts either by telephone or in person.

- Debriefing the team, and untoward incidents reported, particularly equipment or system failures (see below). Audit forms should be completed and this may be carried out by the leader or delegated as appropriate.

Team membership

Wherever possible, the duty team should meet at the beginning of their period on duty to form a 'huddle' as previously described. Any patients who have been identified as 'at risk' during the previous duty period should be reviewed.

Every effort should be made to enable the team members to meet at the end of their duty to debrief (Figure 10.1), to discuss what went well and what could be improved. It may also be possible to carry out a formal handover to the incoming team.

Teamwork is one of the most important non-technical skills that contribute to successful management of critical situations. In a team, the members usually have complementary skills and can coordinate their efforts to work synergistically. There are several characteristics of a good resuscitation team member:

- Competence – has the skills required at a cardiorespiratory arrest and performs them to the best of their ability.

- Commitment – the team has a common goal, the best outcome for the patient.

- Communication – open, indicating their findings and actions taken.

- Communication can be a challenge. A challenge may be cognitive – concerns regarding a diagnosis or safety issue. This can be challenging and team leaders and members should be considerate in their phraseology; in this way can one can challenge a leader without elevating stress for both team leaders and members

Examples:

" I wonder if we should consider the use ...."

" I think we could try........"

" Should we get extra expert help now..?."

" I am happy to lead if you would appreciate the help....."

A good team member:

- listens carefully to briefings and instructions from the team leader

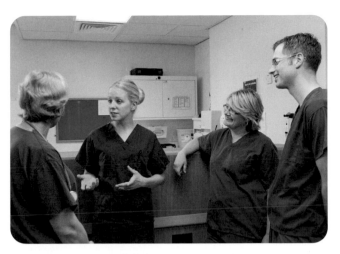

Figure 10.1 Team debrief

- is supportive and facilitative – allows others to achieve their best

- is accountable – for their own and the team's actions and recognises when help is needed

- may be creative, suggesting different ways of interpreting the situation

- participates in providing feedback

- helps the team to maintain situational awareness.

Task management

The many decisions to be made usually fall to the team leader. The leader will assimilate information from the team members, personal observation and will use this to determine appropriate interventions. Typical decisions made include:

- planning and briefing the team, if feasible prior to the arrival of the patient

- sharing the initial plan and delegation of tasks to the team

- diagnosis of the cardiorespiratory arrest rhythm

- choice of shock energy to be used for defibrillation

- likely reversible causes of the cardiorespiratory arrest

- decision making regarding how long to continue resuscitation

- to ensure that decisions have been implemented

- identification of resources required.

Post resuscitation care

Resuscitation does not stop with return of spontaneous circulation (ROSC). Handing the patient over to another colleague, or department or to a different hospital all require good communication and the SBAR or RSVP tool can provide a framework for information sharing at this stage.

High quality care

The Institute of Medicine defines that quality care is safe, effective, patient-centred, timely, efficient and equitable. Hospitals, resuscitation teams and PILS providers should ensure they deliver these aspects of quality to improve the care of the deteriorating patient and patients in cardiorespiratory arrest. Two aspects of this are safety incident reporting (also called adverse or critical incident reporting) and collecting good quality data.

Safety incident reporting

Hospitals now report patient safety incidents to the NHS Commissioning Board Special Health Authority, which ensures patient safety is at the heart of the NHS, previously the domain of the National Patient Safety Agency (NPSA). A patient safety incident is defined as 'any unintended or unexpected incident that could have harmed or did lead to harm for one or more patients being cared for by the National Health Service (NHS). A review of NPSA safety incidents relating to cardiorespiratory arrest and patient deterioration by the Resuscitation Council (UK) shows that the most common reported incidents are associated with equipment problems, communication, delays in the resuscitation team attending and failure to escalate treatment.

Audit and outcome after cardiac arrest

Most modern defibrillators allow the cardiorespiratory arrest management to be downloaded with a time-line of different rhythms and actions taken in terms of defibrillation, cardioversion and cardiopulmonary resuscitation. Locally, this useful information can help teams use reflection and feedback to improve future performance especially in terms of adherence to resuscitation guidelines, the percentage of time CPR has been performed and 'hands-off' time.

National audit of the processes and outcomes provides information about whether interventions and changes made to resuscitation guidelines improve patient care. It is essential the resuscitation outcome and processes are reported in a standard manner to allow comparison between different areas of practice. The internationally agreed Utstein template is a standardised system of reporting that allows the comparison of resuscitation data across different countries and healthcare systems. This facilitates the use of large national and multi-national databases to evaluate the impact of new drugs or techniques.

New interventions that improve survival rate even marginally are important because of the many victims of cardiorespiratory arrest each year. Local hospitals or healthcare systems are unlikely to have sufficient patients to identify these effects or eliminate confounders. One way around this dilemma is by adopting uniform definitions and collecting standardised data on both the process and outcome of resuscitation on many patients in multiple centres. Changes in the resuscitation process can

then be introduced and evaluated using a reliable measure of outcome. This methodology enables drugs and techniques developed in experimental studies to be evaluated reliably in the clinical setting.

In the UK, the National Cardiac Arrest Audit (NCAA) is an ongoing, national, comparative outcome audit of in-hospital cardiac arrests. It is a joint initiative between the Resuscitation Council (UK) and the Intensive Care National Audit & Research Centre (ICNARC) and is open to all acute hospitals in the UK and Ireland. The audit monitors and reports on the incidence of, and outcome from, in-hospital cardiorespiratory arrest in order to inform practice and policy. It aims to identify and foster improvements in the prevention, care delivery and outcomes from cardiorespiratory arrest. Data are collected according to standardised definitions and entered onto the NCAA secure web-based system. Once data are validated, hospitals are provided with activity reports and comparative reports, allowing a comparison of to be made not only within, but also between, hospitals locally, nationally and internationally. Furthermore it also enables the effects of introducing changes to guidelines, new drugs, new techniques etc to be monitored that would not be possible on a hospital-by-hospital basis (Table 10.2).

Table 10.2 Outcomes following in-hospital cardiac arrest (UK) for children in participating hospitals 2015-2017 NCAA data. Total number Cardiac arrests = 1022

	VF/pVT	Asystole	PEA
% of arrests*	4.1%	23.9%	30.7%
% ROSC > 20 mins	74%	37%	66%
% Hospital discharge	72%	25%	47%
Overall survival to hospital discharge	51.1%		

*Remainder cardiac arrests bradycardia or other.

Summary learning

- **Non-technical skills are important during resuscitation.**
- **Use SBAR or RSVP for effective communication.**
- **Report safety incidents and collect cardiac arrest data to help improve patient care.**

My key take-home messages from this chapter

pILS

pILS

		ADRENALINE	FLUID BOLUS	GLUCOSE	SODIUM BICARBONATE		TRACHEAL TUBE UNCUFFED	TRACHEAL TUBE CUFFED	DEFIBRILLATION
STRENGTH		1:10,000	0.9% Saline	10%	4.2%	8.4%			4 joules kg⁻¹
DOSE		10 mcg kg⁻¹	20 mL kg⁻¹	2 mL kg⁻¹	1 mmol kg⁻¹				Trans-thoracic
ROUTE		IV, IO	IV, IO	IV, IO	IV, IO,	IV, IO			Monophasic or biphasic
NOTES			Consider warmed fluids	For known hypoglycaemia. Recheck glucose after dose And repeat as required				Monitor cuff pressure	
AGE	**WEIGHT kg**	mL	mL	mL	mL	mL	ID mm	ID mm	Manual
<1 month	3.5	0.35	70	7	7	-	3.0	-	20
1 month	4	0.4	80	8	8	-	3.0 - 3.5	3.0	20
3 months	5	0.5	100	10	10	-	3.5	3.0	20
6 months	7	0.7	140	14	-	7	3.5	3.0	30
1 year	10	1.0	200	20	-	10	4.0	3.5	40
2 years	12	1.2	240	24	-	12	4.5	4.0	50
3 years	14	1.4	280	28	-	14	4.5 - 5.0	4.0 - 4.5	60
4 years	16	1.6	320	32	-	16	5.0	4.5	60
5 years	18	1.8	360	36	-	18	5.0 - 5.5	4.5 - 5.0	70
6 years	20	2.0	400	40	-	20	5.5	5.0	80
7 years	23	2.3	460	46	-	23	5.5 - 6.0	5.0 - 5.5	100
8 years	26	2.6	500	50	-	26	-	6.0 - 6.5	100
10 years	30	3.0	500	50	-	30	-	7.0	120
12 years	38	3.8	500	50	-	38	-	7 - 7.5	120
14 years	40	4.0	500	50	-	40	-	7 - 8	120 - 150
Adolescent	50kg	5.0	500	50	-	50	-	7 - 8	120 - 150
Adult	70kg	10.0	500	50	-	50	-	7 - 8	120 - 150

Cardioversion — Synchronised Shock – 1.0 joules kg⁻¹ escalating to 2.0 joules kg⁻¹ if unsuccessful.

Amiodarone — 5 mg kg⁻¹ IV or IO bolus in arrest (0.1 mL kg⁻¹ of 150 mg in 3 mL) after 3rd and 5th shocks. Flush line with 0.9% saline or 5% glucose.

Atropine — 20 mcg kg⁻¹, maximum dose 600 mcg.

Calcium chloride 10% — 0.2 mL kg⁻¹ for hypocalcaemia hyperkalaemia.

Lorazepam — 100 mcg kg⁻¹ IV or IO for treatment of seizures. Can be repeated after 10 min. Maximum single dose 4mg.

Adenosine — 100 mcg kg⁻¹ IV or IO for treatment of SVT. Second dose may be doubled requires large saline flush and ECG monitoring.

Anaphylaxis — Adrenaline 1:1000 **intramuscularly** (<6 yrs 150 mcg [0.15 mL], 6-12 yrs 300 mcg [0.3 mL], >12 yrs 500 mcg [0.5mL]) can be repeated after five min.
(**OR** titrate boluses of 1 mcg kg⁻¹ IV **ONLY** if familiar with giving IV adrenaline).

Weights averaged on lean body mass from 50th centile weights for males and females. Drug doses based on Resuscitation Council (UK) Guidelines 2015 recommendations.
Recommendations for tracheal tubes are based on full term neonates.
For newborns glucose at 2.5mL kg⁻¹ is recommended.

Anaphylaxis Algorithm

Anaphylactic reaction?

↓

Airway, Breathing, Circulation, Disability, Exposure

↓

Diagnosis - look for:
- Acute onset of illness
- Life-threatening Airway and/or Breathing and/or Circulation problems [1]
- And usually skin changes

↓

- **Call for help**
- Lie patient flat
- Raise patient's legs

↓

Adrenaline [2]

↓

When skills and equipment available:
- Establish airway
- High flow oxygen
- IV fluid challenge [3]
- Chlorphenamine [4]
- Hydrocortisone [5]

Monitor:
- Pulse oximetry
- ECG
- Blood pressure

---

[1] Life-threatening problems:

Airway:	swelling, hoarseness, stridor
Breathing:	rapid breathing, wheeze, fatigue, cyanosis, SpO_2 < 92%, confusion
Circulation:	pale, clammy, low blood pressure, faintness, drowsy/coma

---

[2] Adrenaline (give IM unless experienced with IV adrenaline)
IM doses of 1:1000 adrenaline (repeat after 5 min if no better)

- Adult   500 micrograms IM (0.5 mL)
- Child more than 12 years: 500 micrograms IM (0.5 mL)
- Child 6 -12 years: 300 micrograms IM (0.3 mL)
- Child less than 6 years: 150 micrograms IM (0.15 mL)

Adrenaline IV to be given **only by experienced specialists**
Titrate: Adults 50 micrograms; Children 1 microgram/kg

[3] IV fluid challenge:

Adult - 500 – 1000 mL
Child - crystalloid 20 mL/kg

Stop IV colloid
if this might be the cause
of anaphylaxis

---

	[4] Chlorphenamine (IM or slow IV)	[5] Hydrocortisone (IM or slow IV)
Adult or child more than 12 years	10 mg	200 mg
Child 6 - 12 years	5 mg	100 mg
Child 6 months to 6 years	2.5 mg	50 mg
Child less than 6 months	250 micrograms/kg	25 mg

Recognition of asthma

These clinical features increase the probability of a diagnosis of asthma:
- More than one of the following: wheeze, cough, difficulty breathing and chest tightness. The risk is increased if these symptoms are recurrent, worse at night or in the early morning, occur during or after exercise or trigger dependent (e.g. with exposure to pets, cold, humidity, heightened emotions or occurring independent of upper respiratory tract infections)
- Personal history of atopic disorder
- Family history of atopic disorder and/or asthma
- Widespread wheeze heard on auscultation
- History of improvement in symptoms or lung function in response to adequate therapy.

Acute asthma in children under 2 years

The assessment of acute asthma in early childhood can be difficult
- Intermittent wheezing attacks are usually due to viral infection and the response to asthma medication is inconsistent
- Prematurity and low birth weight are risk factors for recurrent wheezing
- The differential diagnosis of symptoms includes: – aspiration pneumonitis – pneumonia – bronchiolitis – tracheomalacia – complications of underlying conditions such as congenital anomalies and cystic fibrosis.

Classification of severity of acute presentation

Moderate	Acute Severe	Life-threatening

• Normal mental state
• Ability to talk in sentences or vocalise as normal
• Some accessory muscle use
• PEF ≥ 50% of best or predicted
• O_2 saturations > 92% in air
• Moderate tachycardia
  HR ≤ 125 min^{-1} (> 5 years)
  HR ≤ 140 min^{-1} (2–5 years)
• RR ≤ 30 min^{-1} (> 5 years)
• RR ≤ 40 min^{-1} (2–5 years)
	• Agitated, distressed
	• Can't complete sentences in one breath
	• Moderate to marked accessory muscle use
	• PEF 33–50% of best or predicted
	• O_2 saturations < 92% in air
	• HR > 125 min^{-1} (> 5 years)
	• HR > 140 min^{-1} (2–5 years)
	• RR > 30 min^{-1} (> 5 years)
	• RR > 40 min^{-1} (2–5 years)
		• Confused, drowsy, exhausted
		• Unable to talk
		• Maximal accessory muscle use (poor respiratory effort is pre-terminal)
		• Marked tachycardia (sudden fall in HR is pre-terminal)
		• PEF < 33% of best or predicted
		• O_2 saturations < 92% in air
		• Silent chest
		• Cyanosis
		• Hypotension

Management

Moderate	Acute Severe	Life-threatening
• Continuous O_2 saturation monitoring • High flow O_2 via face mask titrated to achieve O_2 saturations 94–98% • β2 agonist 2–10 puffs via pMDI + spacer +/-facemask, repeat dose every 20 min reviewing effect; no improvement in 1 h treat as acute severe. • Ipratropium bromide given early via pMDI + spacer +/- facemask, particularly if poorly responsive to β2 agonist • Oral steroids: 20 mg prednisolone for children aged 2 to 5 years; 30 to 40 mg for children > 5 years	• Continuous O_2 saturation monitoring • High flow O_2 via face mask titrated to achieve O_2 saturations 94–98% • β2 agonist nebulised (salbutamol 2.5–5mg) every 20 min with Ipratropium bromide (250mcg) for first 2 h; review frequently. • Consider adding magnesium sulphate 150mg to each β2 and Ipratropium bromide nebuliser in the first hour in children with a short duration of acute asthma presenting with oxygen saturations of < 92% • Oral steroids: 20 mg prednisolone for children aged 2 to 5 years; 30 to 40 mg for children > 5 years • Consider aminophylline if child unresponsive to maximal doses of bronchodilators and steroids • Consider ABG if poor response to early treatment	Continuous O_2 saturation monitoring • High flow O_2 via face mask titrated to achieve O_2 saturations 94–98% • Refer to PICU • β2 agonist nebulised (salbutamol 2.5–5mg) every 20 min with Ipratropium bromide (250mcg) for first 2 h; review frequently. • Consider early single bolus dose of intravenous salbutamol where child has responded poorly to inhaled therapy • Oral steroids: 20 mg prednisolone (2 to 5 years); 30 to 40 mg (> 5 years). Repeat dose if vomiting or consider intravenous steroids (hydrocortisone 4 mg kg^{-1} every 4 h) • Consider aminophylline if child unresponsive to maximal doses of bronchodilators and steroids • Intravenous magnesium is a safe but as yet unproven therapy for acute asthma • Consider ABG if poor response to early treatment

pILS

Useful links

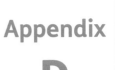

www.resus.org.uk	**Resuscitation Council (UK)**
www.erc.edu	**European Resuscitation Council**
www.ilcor.org	**International Liaison Committee on Resuscitation**
www.americanheart.org	**American Heart Association**
www.nice.org.uk	**The National Institute for Health and Care Excellence (NICE)**
www.rcpch.ac.uk	**Royal College of Paediatrics and Child Health**
www.bhf.org.uk	**British Heart Foundation**
www.ics.ac.uk	**Intensive Care Society**
www.picsociety.uk	**Paediatric Intensive Care Society UK**
www.aagbi.org	**Association of Anaesthetists of Great Britain and Ireland**
www.bestbets.org	**Best evidence topics in emergency medicine**
www.bcs.com	**British Cardiac Society**
www.escardio.org	**European Society of Cardiology**
www.esicm.org	**European Society of Intensive Care Medicine**

 Resuscitation Guidelines   **Resuscitation Council (UK) courses**

 iResus app – easy access to the Resuscitation Guidelines

 Lifesaver app – a new way to learn CPR

 @ResusCouncilUK   **Resuscitation Council UK**   **ResusCouncilUK**